4—

Tamoxifen

A GUIDE
FOR CLINICIANS
AND PATIENTS

Provided through an educational grant
from
Zeneca Pharmaceuticals

Tamoxifen
A GUIDE
FOR CLINICIANS
AND PATIENTS

Edited by V. Craig Jordan, PhD, DSc
Northwestern University Medical School

Note to the reader

The information in this volume has been carefully reviewed for correctness of dosage and indications. Before prescribing any drug, however, the clinician should consult the manufacturer's current package labeling for accepted indications, absolute dosage recommendations, and other information pertinent to the safe and effective use of the product described. This is especially important when drugs are given in combination or as an adjunct to other forms of therapy. Furthermore, some of the medications described, as well as some of the indications mentioned, may not have been approved by the US Food and Drug Administration at the time of publication. This possibility should be borne in mind before prescribing or recommending any drug or regimen.

Library of Congress 96-071318

ISBN 9641823-4-3

For information on obtaining additional copies of this volume,
contact the publishers, PRR, Inc., 17 Prospect Street, Huntington, NY 11743.

H U N T I N G T O N
N E W   Y O R K

Publishers of
ONCOLOGY
Oncology News International
Primary Care & Cancer
Medical Oncology
Cancer Management:
A Multidisciplinary Approach
Myths and Facts About Cancer

"This is not the end, it is not even the beginning of the end.
But it is perhaps the end of the beginning."
Winston Spencer Churchill, 1942

This book is dedicated to the women in my family,
Cynthia, Helen, Alexandra, Monica, Jill, Maxine and Becky
(listed in the order we first met)

Contributors

V. Craig Jordan, PhD, DSc
Director
Breast Cancer Research Program
Robert H. Lurie Cancer Center
Northwestern University Medical School
Chicago

Vasilios J. Assikis, MD
Research Fellow
Robert H. Lurie Cancer Center
Northwestern University Medical School
Chicago

Richard R. Barakat, MD
Assistant Attending Surgeon
Gynecology Service
Memorial Sloan-Kettering Cancer Center
New York

Malcolm M. Bilimoria, MD
Research Fellow
Breast Cancer Research Program
Robert E. Lurie Cancer Center
Northwestern University Medical School
Chicago

Nancy Brinker
Founding Chairwoman
Susan G. Komen Breast Cancer
 Foundation
Dallas

I. Craig Henderson, MD
Adjunct Professor of Medicine
University of California
San Francisco

Amy S. Langer
Executive Director
National Alliance of Breast Cancer
 Organizations (NABCO)
New York

Monica Morrow, MD
Director
Lynn Sage Comprehensive Breast
 Program
Northwestern University Medical School
Chicago

Ruth O'Regan, MD
Fellow
Hematology/Oncology Division
Robert E. Lurie Cancer Center
Northwestern University Medical School
Chicago

C. Kent Osborne, MD
AB Alexander Distinguished Chair
 and Chief of Medical Oncology
University of Texas Health Science Center
San Antonio

Joseph Ragaz, MD
Senior Medical Oncologist
Vancouver Cancer Centre
British Columbia Cancer Agency
University of British Columbia
Vancouver

Peter M. Ravdin, MD
Associate Professor of Medicine/
 Oncology
University of Texas Health Science Center
San Antonio

Norman Wolmark, MD
Chairman
National Surgical Adjuvant Breast and
 Bowel Project (NSABP)

Chairman
Department of Human Oncology
Medical College of Pennsylvania/
 Hahnemann University
Allegheny Campus
Pittsburgh

About the Author and Editor

Although Professor Jordan is only one of the many who have contributed to the successful development of tamoxifen, his credentials for writing and editing this book are unique. He has been involved in the research and development of antiestrogens for more than a quarter of a century and has been a strong advocate for

V. Craig Jordan

the clinical evaluation of tamoxifen. His work in the early 1970s promoted the development of ICI46,474 from a laboratory curiosity to its position today as the world's most important drug for the treatment of breast cancer and the most frequently prescribed cancer therapy. Specifically, Professor Jordan formulated the concepts of prevention and long-term adjuvant therapy in the laboratory and successfully translated these ideas to clinical trials and clinical practice.

Professor Jordan has served on the editorial board, as associate or managing editor, of more than ten scientific and medical journals, including *Breast Cancer Research and Treatment, Cancer Letters, Cancer Research, Clinical Cancer Research, European Journal of Cancer, Journal of the National Cancer Institute*, and *ONCOLOGY*.

To mark his contributions to medicine, Professor Jordan has received numerous prestigious national and international awards. In 1989, Professor Jordan and Professor Lerner, the scientist who discovered the first nonsteroidal antiestrogen, MER25, jointly received the Eighth Bruce F. Cain Memorial Award from the American Association for Cancer Research for "outstanding preclinical research in cancer chemotherapy." In 1992, Professor Jordan received the Inaugural Brinker International Award for Basic Research in Breast Cancer from the Susan G. Komen Foundation in Dallas. The award was presented in the presence of the Vice President of the United States. The following year, Professor Jordan received the American Society for Pharmacology and Experimental Therapeutics Award for research on human disease and the Sir John Gaddum Award at Cambridge University, England, from the British Pharmacological Society for his important contributions to pharmacology.

Most importantly, in 1993, Professor Jordan was selected to receive the Cameron prize from the University of Edinburgh. Recipients of this award are a select group of medical researchers from any field who have changed the practice of therapeutics. The 100 awardees are considered to have made the most important medical contributions in the world during the past century.

Recently, Professor Jordan was selected as the recipient of the American-Italian Award for Scientific Excellence in Medicine for his research contributions towards the prevention of breast cancer (1995) and of the Block Award for Distinguished Achievement in Cancer Research by Ohio State University (1996).

Contents

continued on the following page

Contents *continued*

Nancy Brinker

Foreword

Tamoxifen has changed the treatment of breast cancer and brought hope to the millions of women who develop the disease. Tamoxifen was first introduced in the United States in 1978. Although it was originally indicated for the treatment of advanced disease in postmenopausal women, since then the Food and Drug Administration has approved the expanded use of tamoxifen for the treatment of all stages of breast cancer. However, this remarkable drug was only developed to its full potential by dedicated research ventures that ultimately has made such a profound difference in so many women's lives.

At the Komen Foundation, we are dedicated to the goal of finding a cure for breast cancer through research. To achieve our goal, we are pledged to raise the financial resources to conduct first-class laboratory and clinical research in our nation's finest universities and cancer centers. It is people who make discoveries and who change our understanding of breast cancer. We are, therefore, committed to defeating breast cancer by providing fellowships for the best and the brightest young doctors and scientists to start their careers in centers of scientific excellence. The Komen Foundation is pleased to have supported research on tamoxifen in Dr. Jordan's laboratories at the University of Wisconsin (Madison) and Northwestern University in Chicago, and in Dr. Osborne's laboratory at the University of Texas in San Antonio. Both doctors are contributors to this book.

We also strongly believe that successes in research should be recognized, because these are milestones by which we can measure our progress. In 1992, to mark the 10th anniversary of the Susan G. Komen Foundation, we established the Brinker International Breast Cancer Award for completed research. A blue-ribbon panel of scientists and doctors was charged with selecting a recipient for the Inaugural Brinker International Breast Cancer Award for Basic Research. The committee selected Dr. V. Craig Jordan for his dedication to breast cancer research and for guiding the successful clinical development of tamoxifen. The citation reads, "Dr. Jordan has been tireless in his sustained effort to provide underlying scientific strategies for the clinical value of tamoxifen which has resulted in improved survival for thousands of women with primary breast cancer."

The success of tamoxifen is the result of a close collaboration between Zeneca Pharmaceuticals, the agent's discoverer and manufacturer, and the academic and clinical communities. Tamoxifen is the first clinically useful antiestrogen for breast cancer treatment, and its widespread use has changed the way breast cancer is treated. The beneficiaries of the successful research and progress that are described in this book, by the doctors and scientists who made the discoveries, are the millions of women with breast cancer. Tamoxifen represents a successful battle in the war we are waging against breast cancer. Only through cooperation, research, and advancing knowledge can we look forward to a brighter future when breast cancer has been conquered.

Nancy Brinker
Founding Chairwoman
Susan G. Komen Breast Cancer Foundation

Acknowledgments,
With Five Photo Collages

On the following pages you will find photographs of the many investigators and clinicians, friends and colleagues who were important in the discovery and development of tamoxifen. The author wishes to acknowledge their most important contributions to the research in the field of antiestrogens.

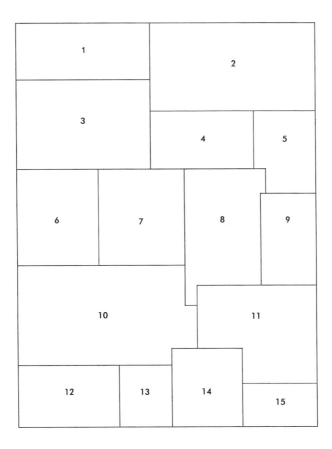

1. **L to R: Alex Pleuvry, Dr. John Patterson** (who had recently joined ICI), and the author at the International Congress of Chemotherapy, London 1975. Dr. Patterson became responsible at ICI for coordinating clinical trials with Nolvadex, notably the NATO Trial.

2. **L to R: Drs. Douglas Tormey** then head of the Breast Cancer Committee of ECOG, the author, Anna Reigel (nee Tate) and Paul Carbone, Chairman of ECOG, Wisconsin, 1983.

3. **Drs. Geof Greene (l) and the late Bill McGuire (r)**, International Congress of Chemotherapy, Budapest, 1986. Dr. Greene developed monoclonal antibodies to the estrogen receptor and Dr. McGuire developed the concept of the progesterone receptor as a prognostic indicator.

4. **Michael Baum**, Professor of Surgery at the Royal Marsden Hospital, London and his wife Judy, attending an International Breast Cancer meeting in Florida, 1991.

5. **Dr. C. Kent Osborne**, Head of Medical Oncology, University of Texas, San Antonio, at a breast cancer meeting in Colorado, 1987. He is internationally recognized for his research on tamoxifen resistance and the treatment of hormone dependent breast cancer.

6. **Professor Keith Griffith** (Director of the Tenovus Institute for Cancer Research, Cardiff, Wales) and Dr. Rob Nicholson, at an estrogen receptor meeting in Monte Carlo, 1984. Dr. Nicholson completed some of the first laboratory studies of tamoxifen as an antitumor agent in the United Kingdom.

7. **Drs. Benita Katzenellenbogen and Henri Rochefort**, Steroid Biochemistry meeting, Canary Isles, 1989. Both scientists have provided invaluable knowledge to our understanding of the basic aspects of estrogen and antiestrogen action.

8. **Drs. Gerald Mueller**, Lasker Professor of Oncology, Jack Gorski, Professor of Biochemistry and Harold Rusch, founding director of the McArdle Laboratory and the Wisconsin Clinical Cancer Center, Wisconsin, 1985.

9. **Professor Manfred Kaufman**, Chairman, Department of Gynecology, University of Heidelberg at a breast cancer meeting in Japan, 1994. Professor Kaufman has completed pivotal studies of Zoladex for the treatment of breast cancer in premenopausal women.

10. **L to R: the author, Dr. Norman Wolmark**, now the Chairman of the NSABP, **Professor O. Abe**, our host, **Professor Michael Baum**, Chairman of NATO **and Professor John Forbes**, Chairman, Breast Committee, Australia and New Zealand Oncology Group at a breast cancer meeting in Japan, 1986.

11. **Lois Trench-Hines** receiving an award from Dr. Paul Carbone, at a breast cancer meeting in Florida, 1991, for her commitment to the early development of Nolvadex.

12. **Dr. Bernard Fisher**, then Chairman of the NSABP, with Mrs. Louise Rusch on the occasion of the inaugural Rusch Memorial Breast Cancer Lecture, 1991. As chairman of the NSABP, Dr. Fisher laid the foundation for current standards of breast cancer treatment in the United States.

13. **Professor Roger Blamey**, Chairman of Surgery at Nottingham City Hospital, England, 1990. He has completed pivotal studies with Zoladex and the new pure antiestrogen in women with breast cancer.

14. **Dr. Trevor Powles**, Director of the Breast Cancer Program at the Royal Marsden Hospital, London, attending the Miami International Breast Cancer Conference, 1995. He initiated the first pilot prevention study with tamoxifen in 1986.

15. **Dr. Richard Love**, organizer of the Wisconsin Tamoxifen Study that showed that tamoxifen maintains bone density in postmenopausal women, and the author, on a visit to England, 1988.

Acknowledgments

This book began as the result of conversations with hundreds of women with breast cancer who wanted to learn more about tamoxifen. I owe a great debt of gratitude to each one of these women for the help and insight they provided. Most importantly, without the constant support and encouragement of my wife Monica, the manuscript for this book could not have been finished. I thank Jack Gentile and Jim McCarthy of PRR Publishers for their support in organizing the Tamoxifen Roundtable held in San Antonio in December 1995, and to the participants and contributors for making this project a success.

I especially thank Nancy Brinker for agreeing to contribute the Foreword for my book, as well as Sharon Green and Michelle Melin of Y-Me in Chicago for help in identifying patients' specific concerns about tamoxifen.

I must thank the more than 70 staff, students, and fellows of the "tamoxifen teams," who, over the past 25 years, have translated ideas into results in my laboratories in England, Switzerland, and the United States. Special thanks must also go to my many colleagues at ICI Pharmaceuticals (now, Zeneca), whose friendship and support transformed laboratory concepts into clinical benefits.

Rather than list all the names of my friends and colleagues who have made possible the successes of the past 28 years, I have chosen to acknowledge their contributions in the five photographic collages shown in this section.

Finally, I thank my secretary, Susan Tripoli, for patiently typing (and retyping) the numerous versions of the manuscript; Henry Muenzner for completing some of the figures; Dr. Michael Dukes of Zeneca for locating the pictures of the Queens Award for Technological Achievement, and Dr. Dora Richardson. Jim Ziv deserves a special thanks for taking the photograph on the dedication page and the one of my current laboratory.

This book would not have been published without the tireless efforts of the editorial/art/production team at PRR: Craig Falzone, Jeannine Coronna, Lisa Katz, Lois Friedman, Stacey Zebrowski, Gail van Koot, Andy Nash, Mia Lipp, Roseanne Szczepanowski, Madeline McCarthy, and Joan Deters. I owe each person a great debt of gratitude for their dedication to this project.

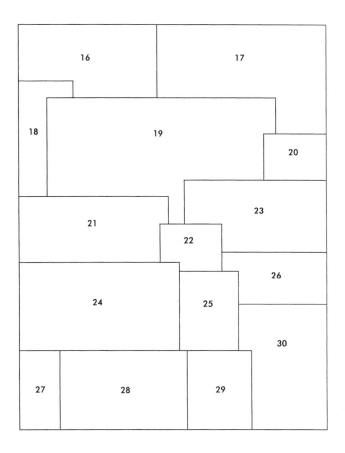

16. **Some of the attendees at the Bill McGuire Memorial Dinner** at the Langston House, New Braunfels, Texas, 1994. L to R: Dr. Gary Clark, Biostatistician who developed the concept of prognosticators for breast cancer, Mini DeLaGarza, Administrative Assistant to Bill McGuire and Dr. Peter Ravdin, Associate Professor of Oncology, University of Texas, San Antonio (former Tamoxifen Team member).

17. **Tamoxifen Team, 1986**, University of Wisconsin. Back row L to R: Dawn Mirecki, Cathy Murphy, Ethel Cormier, Dave Whitford, Nancy Fritz, Marco Gottardis, Mary Janes, Mike Wolf, Richard Bain, Eric Phelps, Pat Morton. Front Row, Simon Robinson, Wade Welshons, the author, Peter Ravdin, Rick Koch.

18. **Professor R. Charles Coombes, MD**, Chairman of Medical Oncology, Charing Cross Hospital, London, visiting Madison, Wisconsin, 1984. Dr. Coombes did the first clinical studies with the aromatase inhibitor discovered by the Brodies at the Worcester Foundation (#46 and #74).

19. **Tamoxifen Team, 1991**, at the International Antihormones in Breast Cancer meeting Orlando, Florida.

20. **Dr. Doug Wolf**, former PhD student, 1992. He discovered a natural point mutation of the estrogen receptor in a tamoxifen-stimulated tumor, and described a new model to explain how adjuvant tamoxifen therapy might work.

21. **American Association for Cancer Research Meeting,** B.F. Cain Award Reception, 1989. L to R: Drs. Simon Robinson, Cathy Murphy, the author, Ethel Cormier, Marco Gottardis.

22. **Mike Fritsch, MD, PhD,** currently working at the National Institutes of Health, Washington. He obtained his Doctor of Philosophy with Jack Gorski and was a postdoctoral fellow in the author's laboratory, 1991. He originally worked with Dr. Mara Lieberman and has conducted numerous studies on the estrogen receptor and antiestrogen action.

23. **ICI Pharmaceuticals, Alderley Park, 1986.** Alan Wakeling, discoverer of the pure antiestrogens, Alex Pleuvry, responsible for global marketing of Nolvadex, Barry Furr, the Director of Bioscience II and responsible for the development of Zoladex and Casodex and Sandy Todd, Product Development Manager.

24. **Madrid, 1986.** Steroid Biochemistry Meeting. L to R: Drs. Roger King, who has provided fundamental insights into hormone-dependent and independent tumor growth, the author, and Rob Sutherland, who is recognized for the basic understanding of estrogen and antiestrogen action in the cell cycle.

25. **Dr. Michael Gould,** Professor of Human Oncology, University of Wisconsin, 1993. Responsible for discovering new natural products as breast cancer preventives currently being tested by Professor Coombes. (#18)

26. **B.F. Cain Memorial Award Dinner, 1989.** Dr. Syd Salmon, Director of the Arizona Cancer Center and his wife Joannie. In the center is Dr. Len Lerner, the discoverer of the first nonsteroidal antiestrogen MER 25 and the fertility drug clomiphene.

27. **The late Dr. Olaf Pearson,** Case Western Reserve, at a breast cancer meeting in Madison, Wisconsin, 1984. Dr. Pearson did some of the first work on adrenal estrogen and was among the first to test tamoxifen in the United States.

28. **Graduation, University of Wisconsin, 1991.** Dr. Shun-Yuan Jiang, who created new breast cancer cell lines with the re-introduction of the estrogen receptor gene and is now an Associate Professor in Taiwan, the author, and Amy Stella.

29. **Professor Adrian Harris,** Oxford University, at the St. Galen Breast Cancer Meeting, Switzerland, 1992. Professor Harris has used antiestrogens to reverse chemotherapeutic drug resistance and is recognized for his work on angiogenesis.

30. **Partial Tamoxifen Team, 1989**: Back Row L to R: Chris Parker, Mary Lababidi, Mark Thompson, John Pink. Front Row: Marco Gottardis, Cathy Murphy.

Collage Number 3, composed of photos 31 through 43,

appears on the following page

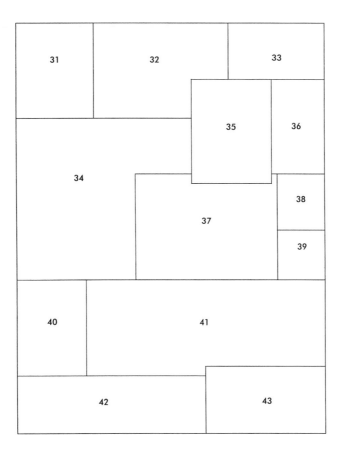

31. **Dr. John Katzenellenbogen**, Professor of Chemistry, University of Illinois, Madison, Meeting on Antiestrogens and Estrogens, 1984. His skill as an organic chemist has proved to be invaluable for the synthesis and identification of estrogens and antiestrogens. The biological studies were completed with his wife, Benita (see #7).

32. **Center: Dr. Marc Lippman**, Director of the Vincent T. Lombardi Cancer Center, Washington, DC; the Inaugural Lynn Sage Visiting Professor, 1995. His research program for the past 25 years has provided fundamental links between hormones and growth factors and he has mapped out future biological strategies for breast cancer therapy.

33. **Professor Yuchi Iino**, Gunma University, Japan, 1993. A former member of the Tamoxifen Team (1988-89).

34. **The Tamoxifen Team, 1983**. Back Row L to R: Stewart Lyman, Dawn Mirecki, Marco Gottardis, Ethel Cormier, Richard Bain, Eric Phelps, the author, the late Dr. Mara Lieberman.

35. **Dr. Edward R. Clark** (my PhD Supervisor, 1969-72), formerly of the Department of Pharmacology, University of Leeds. Pictured at the Gaddum Memorial Award Ceremony, Cambridge University, 1993.

36. **Dr. Henry Pitot**, former Director of the McArdle Laboratory, University of Wisconsin. He is one of the leading authorities on rat liver carcinogenesis and has contributed important new data on the effects of antiestrogens.

37. **The author and Dr. Timothy Jaspan** (then a medical student). Open Day, University of Leeds Medical School, 1976. He is now a consultant physician in Nottingham, United Kingdom. He did some of the early studies of tamoxifen and breast tumor growth in the author's laboratory in 1975.

38. **Professor Rob Sutherland**, Garvin Institute, Sydney, Australia. His distinguished career has resulted in the description of cellular antiestrogen binding sites, the reason for "tumor flare" with antiestrogen treatment, and the interaction of progestins and antiestrogens in the cell cycle.

39. **Dr. David Gibson**, postdoctoral fellow (1988-1990). He is a former member of the Tamoxifen Team who did the first studies to show that tamoxifen plus interferon can completely control breast cancer growth under laboratory conditions.

40. **Dr. Andreas Friedl**, a visiting fellow from Germany in 1988 and now in the Department of Pathology, University of Wisconsin. A former member of the Tamoxifen Team who completed unique studies about hormone responsive tumor growth of hormone-independent cancer cells in animals.

41. **Tamoxifen Team**, Northwestern University, 1996. Back Row L to R: Dr. Claudia Tellez, Henry Muenzner, Dr. Zehan Chen, Dr. Malcolm Bilimoria, Dr. Anna Levenson, Dr. Vasilios Assikis. Front Row L to R: Kala Tanjiori, the author, Dr. Debra Tonetti, Angela Cisneros, Jennifer MacGregor, Julie Yang.

42. **L to R: Douglas Tormey, Franco Cavali**, (Helen Jordan, age 11), **Henri Rochefort** (rear), **Geof Greene, Norman Wolmark, the author, Gene DeSombre**, Madison, Wisconsin, 1984.

43. **Professor Umberto Veronesi**, Scientific Director of the European Institute of Oncology, Milan and Dr. Gabriel Hortobagyi, Chairman, Breast and Gynecologic Cancers, M.D. Anderson Cancer Center, Houston, Texas, 1995. Professor Veronesi has championed the use of conservative surgery as a treatment for breast cancer and published the first studies showing the value of the approach.

Captions for this collage are on the next page ▶

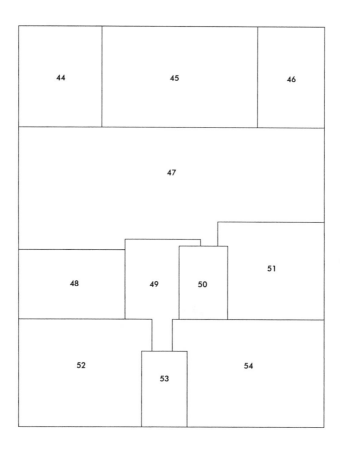

44. **Dr. Donald ("Skip") Trump, 1986.** He has organized clinical studies to evaluate high-dose tamoxifen as a strategy to combat drug resistance to chemotherapy. He is currently Director for Clinical Research at the University of Pittsburgh.

45. **The remainder of the current Tamoxifen Team** at Northwestern University Medical School, Robert H. Lurie Cancer Center (see #41). Dr. Gale England, Michael Piette and Dr. Ruth O'Regan.

46. **Dr. Angela Brodie, Hamburg, 1987.** She is currently Professor of Pharmacology at the University of Maryland and with her husband Harry completed the first laboratory studies on the antitumor use of 4-hydroxyandrostenedione at the Worcester Foundation, 1974-76 (see #74).

47. **The European School of Oncology** Breast Cancer Task Force, Italy, 1986. Dr. Frances Cavali, the chairman, is seated at the front. On the left of the author is Dr. Peter Walton (Zeneca) and the right is Dr. Aron Goldhirsch chairman of the International Breast Cancer Study Group. Behind Dr. Simon Soez (lady seated right) is Dr. Henig Mowidsen from Denmark who completed numerous clinical studies with tamoxifen.

48. **The Tamoxifen Team** remaining at the University of Wisconsin, 1993-95. Matt Bong, Dr. Bill Catherino, who provided a valuable insight into the molecular biology

of tamoxifen resistance, Jim Holson and Dr. John Pink who identified the first high molecular weight estrogen receptor and described the loss of estrogen receptors in breast cancer cells.

49. **Mary Lababidi, 1990.** She ran the steroid receptor laboratory at the University of Wisconsin Comprehensive Cancer Center that serves Southern Wisconsin. She also completed the animal studies to demonstrate that tamoxifen prevents mammary cancer in mice.

50. **Dr. Bill Gradishar,** Medical Oncologist in the Breast Cancer Program at Northwestern University, who has completed several recent clinical reviews of new antiestrogens with the author (see Appendix 6).

51. **Dr. Anna Riegel,** a graduate of the Department of Pharmacology and Steroid Endocrinology at the University of Leeds in the 1970s. She came to America as a Fulbright Hays Scholar to complete her PhD at the McArdle Laboratory in Wisconsin. She was the first member of the Tamoxifen Team in the U.S. in 1980 and described differences between estrogen receptors bound to estradiol or 4-hydroxytamoxifen. She is currently Associate Professor of Pharmacology at Georgetown University in Washington, D.C.

52. **Professor Elwood Jensen and his wife** at a General Motors Prize dinner in Washington. Professor Jensen did the pioneering studies to identify the estrogen receptor and in the late 1960s devised the estrogen receptor assay to predict the hormone responsiveness of breast cancer. In parallel studies with Jack Gorski's group (see #8), he developed models of estrogen action and subsequently isolated the receptor to make monoclonal antibodies that are used in clinical assays today. Dr. Gene DeSombre was Professor Jensen's co-investigator throughout the late 1960s and 70s (#42). Dr. Geof Greene (#3) is the immunologist who trained with Professor Jensen and conducted the laboratory investigation to prepare antibodies. Professor Jensen was the Director of the Ben May Laboratory for Cancer Research at the University of Chicago, the Medical Director of the Ludwig Institute for Cancer Research in Switzerland, and is currently a Professor at the Institute for Hormone and Fertility Research in Hamburg, Germany.

53. **Dr. John Patterson** who is currently Territorial Business Director for Zeneca Pharmaceuticals, Alderley Park, United Kingdom.

54. **Dr. Steven Rosen,** Director of the Robert H. Lurie Cancer Center and his wife Candy. Dr. Monica Morrow (r) is Director of the Lynn Sage Comprehensive Breast Center at Northwestern University Medical School and Northwestern Memorial Hospital.

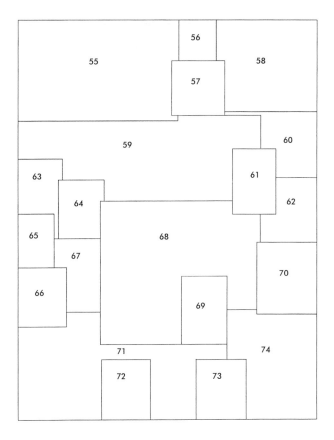

55. **L to R: Drs. Mike Dukes, Barry Furr, and Alan Wakeling**, Zeneca, Macclesfield England, 1996. Alan discovered the pure antiestrogen ICI182,780 and Mike Dukes has been intimately involved in the drug development. Barry Furr has published reviews with the author on tamoxifen and he was specifically involved with the development of Zoladex and Casodex.

56. **Graham Prestwich**, 1977, when he was a research assistant at Leeds University. He is now National Health Trust Accounts Manager for Astra Pharmaceuticals in the North of England.

57. **Dr. Clive Dix** in 1978. He was an ICI Scholar completing his PhD with the author. He described the actions of tamoxifen as an antitumor agent in rats and he defined the pharmacology of 4-hydroxytamoxifen. He is now Director of Research and Development (UK) with Glaxo Wellcome in England.

58. The late **Dr. Jean Bowler**, who synthesized the pure antiestrogens, **and Dr. Brian Newbould**, who was Research Director at ICI (Zeneca) during the late 1970s.

59. **Tamoxifen (Women's) Team 1983**, University of Wisconsin. In the center is Barbara Gosden, who completed some of the first laboratory studies to define antiestrogens with a high affinity for the estrogen receptor. Successor compounds like raloxifene are being tested as preventives for osteoporosis.

60. **Dr. Tony Howell**, a leading medical oncologist at the Christie Hospital, Manchester, England. He has completed the first clinical studies with a pure antiestrogen to define its value as a second therapy after tamoxifen.

61. **Dr. Yvonne Dragan**, McArdle Laboratory, University of Wisconsin. She has completed essential work to define the safety of different antiestrogens. She is working in collaboration with the author and Dr. Henry Pitot (see #36).

62. **Dr. Timothy Kinsella**, Chairman of the Department of Human Oncology, University of Wisconsin.

63. **Graham Prestwich**, the author's research assistant at Leeds University (1974-1977) where we described the first studies with radioactive tamoxifen and estrogen receptor binding and he was part of the team that discovered the potent activity of tamoxifen metabolite 4-hydroxytamoxifen.

64. **Dr. Edward Clark** (1971), the author's PhD supervisor at Leeds University (1969-72). The topic was the structure activity relationships of antiestrogens.

65. **Susan Koerner Ravatoy**, the author's research assistant at the Worcester Foundation (1972-74). We completed the first laboratory studies with tamoxifen as an antitumor agent. She is now involved in genetics testing in New York State.

66. **Susan Lagan-Fahey**, tamoxifen team during the late 1980s at Wisconsin. She was responsible for tamoxifen determinations in long term adjuvant patients and other laboratory studies.

67. **Dr. Kathy Pritchard**, a leading medical oncologist at Sunnybrook, Toronto, Canada. Her clinical work defined the value of tamoxifen both as an adjuvant therapy and as a treatment for premenopausal women.

68. **Dr. Meei-Huey-Jeng** (PhD with the author in 1992), who completed studies linking progestins with breast cancer stimulation. She is now Research Assistant Professor at the University of Virginia. **Dr. Marco Gottardis** (PhD with the author in 1989) was responsible for describing laboratory models of tamoxifen-stimulated tumor growth and for the first studies to show the application of pure antiestrogens as a second line therapy. He is now Senior Research Scientist at Ligand Pharmaceuticals in California.

69. **Dr. Norman Wolmark**, Chairman of the NSABP.

70. **Dr. Guy LeClerq**, Institute Jules Bordet, Brussels, who has completed extensive studies on the antitumor and receptor binding properties of antiestrogens.

71. **The author with David Kupfer**, who has completed pivotal research on the metabolism of tamoxifen, at the Worcester Foundation, 1976.

72. **Dr. Alberto Costa**, Director of the European School of Oncology and one of the organizers of the Italian study to test the worth of tamoxifen as a preventive.

73. **Dr. Harry Brodie**, who started studies (with his wife Angela (picture #46)) on aromatase inhibitors at the Worcester Foundation, 1974.

74. **Dr. Trevor Powles**, the 1992 recipient of the Harold Rusch Memorial Breast Cancer Award with **Mrs. Louise Rusch**, Madison, Wisconsin.

Preface and Introduction

Foundations

V. Craig Jordan, PhD, DSc
Director, Breast Cancer Research Program
Robert H. Lurie Cancer Center
Northwestern University Medical School

In 1967, I met three scientists at ICI Pharmaceuticals Ltd. (now Zeneca) in Cheshire, England who would alter the course of my life and start my involvement in the development of drugs for the treatment of breast cancer. At the time, I was working as a summer student with Dr. Steven Carter, who headed the anticancer screening program, and my project was to study an exciting new natural product, called cytochalasin B, that causes nuclear extrusion from the cell . The compound had no potential as an anticancer agent, but it subsequently found universal use in the laboratory as a tool in cell biology. Twenty years later, Dr. Wade Welshons, working in Dr. Jack Gorski's laboratory and later in my laboratory at the University of Wisconsin, would use the compound to demonstrate that the estrogen receptor was a nuclear protein.

Dr. Arthur Walpole (Figure 1) worked in the laboratory across the corridor from Steven Carter and was head of Reproduction Research. He had just published work on a new antiestrogen, ICI 46,474, that was a potent post-coital contraceptive in the rat. Although there was enormous potential for a new agent to regulate fertility, it was also recognized that antiestrogens could be used to treat breast cancer. This was one of Dr. Walpole's interests.

In the laboratory next to Carter's was Dr. Michael Barrett, then in charge of developing new heart drugs as part of the cardiovascular program. He was responsible for the discovery of practolol and Tenormin. When he became chairman five years later, in 1972, Barrett offered me a faculty position in the Department of Pharmacology at the University of Leeds, and suggested Dr. Arthur Walpole as the external examiner for my PhD on antiestrogens entitled "Structure Activity Relationships of Some Substituted Triphenylethylenes and Triphenylethanols."

In 1969, I had decided to study the estrogen receptor with Dr. Edward Clark in the Department of Pharmacology at the University of Leeds, supported by a research scholarship from the Medical Research Council. Dr.

FIGURE I   Dr. Arthur L. Walpole, who died suddenly on July 2, 1977   At the time of his death he had retired as Head of the Fertility Control Program at ICI's Pharmaceuticals Division in Alderley Park, near Macclesfield, Cheshire but he had continued to work as a consultant on the Joint Research Scheme between ICI and the Department of Pharmacology at the University of Leeds, England.

Jack Gorski had published an exciting series of reports showing that the estrogen receptor could be easily extracted from the rat uterus and isolated by sucrose density gradient analysis. My project was going to be simple. I was to establish the new technique of sucrose density gradient analysis, isolate the receptor, and crystallize the protein with an estrogen and an antiestrogen. Through x-ray crystallography in the Astbury Department of Biophysics at the University of Leeds we would then establish the three-dimensional shape of the complexes to explain antiestrogenic action. The goal was to solve a fundamental question in pharmacology: what is the molecular mechanism of action for a drug? Progress was slow in establishing the receptor purification technique of sucrose gradient analysis, so I switched my thesis topic to study the structure activity relationships of antiestrogens. As it turned out, this was a good strategic decision, as all subsequent attempts by the research community to complete this project have so far met with failure!

In 1972, there was little academic interest in the pharmacology of antiestrogens. Enthusiasm in the pharmaceutical industry had chilled because these drugs had not fulfilled their promise as "morning after" pills. It was clear that no one was recommending antiestrogen research as a sound career choice; it was perceived as a dead end. To make matters worse, the University of Leeds encountered difficulty in securing a qualified examiner for my thesis. Sir Charles Dodds, the discoverer of the synthetic estrogen diethylstilbestrol (DES), declined, with regrets, because he had not to kept up with the literature during the 20 years since his retirement! This situation led Professor Barrett to select Dr. Arthur Walpole from ICI and thus, indirectly, opened the door for the further development of ICI 46,474 to tamoxifen.

When I accepted my faculty position at the University of Leeds in 1972, I was first required to obtain additional research experience elsewhere before I took up my appointment. Professor Barrett solved this problem by arranging for me to work with Dr. Michael Harper at the Worcester Foundation for Experimental Biology in Massachusetts (Figure 2). Dr. Harper is a reproductive biologist who some years earlier had worked with Arthur Walpole at ICI. He is also the co-patent holder for ICI 46,474. However, at that time, Dr. Harper was heading a team at the Foundation working on the potential of prostaglandins to be used as a "once-a-month" contraceptive pill.

When I arrived at the Worcester Foundation in September 1972—incidentally, not knowing anything about prostaglandins—I discovered that Dr. Harper had accepted a job with the World Health Organization in Geneva.

FIGURE 2 **Dr. Michael J. K. Harper, co-patent holder for ICI 46,474.** He discovered the opposing biological activities of the *cis* and *trans* isomers of substituted triphenylethylenes. On the left is Dr. Harper in the mid-1960s, and on the right, on the occasion of his 60th birthday.

My new boss, Dr. Ed Klaiber, said I could do anything I liked as long as some of my work included prostaglandins. I immediately found myself as an independent investigator and I planned my work on prostaglandins. However, my new circumstances would also allow me to explore my passion—to develop a drug for breast cancer.

Beginning the Development of ICI 46,474

Although by 1971 ICI 46,474 had shown modest activity in a preliminary clinical study for the treatment of advanced breast cancer, it was clear that much remained to be done to develop antiestrogens as acceptable therapeutic agents. ICI did not have a breast cancer research program, but Dr. Walpole agreed to help with my request for assistance to conduct a systematic laboratory study of the antitumor properties of tamoxifen at the Worcester Foundation. I had no experience, however, with laboratory models of breast cancer. Fortunately, the Worcester Foundation was a marvelous place to learn as well as find help in new areas of scientific endeavor. Dr. Elwood Jensen, then the director of the Ben May Laboratory for Cancer Research in Chicago, was a member of the scientific advisory board for the Foundation and generously agreed to help me prepare for my study of tamoxifen. The short time I spent in his laboratory, with the help of Dr. Gene DeSombre, was exceptional and provided me with the skills to evaluate the antitumor actions of tamoxifen back in Massachusetts.

To facilitate progress, Dr. Walpole suggested I contact Ms. Lois Trench, the clinical drug monitor for tamoxifen at one of ICI's companies in Wilmington, Delaware. Lois is full of energy and drive and we began a friendship that continues to this day. She admitted that, unfortunately, no one knew much about the new drug in the US clinical department, and she insisted that I become a consultant to encourage clinical trials with tamoxifen. She also arranged for me to study the interaction of tamoxifen with the estrogen receptor and, in 1974, to explain the antitumor effects of tamoxifen at meetings of the Eastern Cooperative Oncology Group (ECOG). Lois subsequently invited me to introduce tamoxifen to the National Surgical Adjuvant Breast and Bowel Project (NSABP) at an international symposium she organized in 1976 in Key Biscayne, Florida.

The work at the Worcester Foundation went exceptionally well. Lois Trench supplied human breast tumors to resolve the controversy of whether tamoxifen inhibited the binding of estrogens to the human estrogen receptor. The first laboratory studies of tamoxifen as a breast cancer preventive were successfully completed in 1974 and Lois sponsored me to present the work at the International Congress of Steroidal Hormones meeting in Mexico City.

There was little interest in the concept at that point (it was 10 years too early!) but, most important, a series of papers was started that fully described the antitumor effects of tamoxifen in animals. Some of that work was included in the handbook given to clinicians in America to support their clinical studies in 1974. The work was also used to support licensing of tamoxifen in Japan and Germany. However, I felt no urgency to publish the results since there was no particular interest in antiestrogens. Contributing to the clinical development of tamoxifen was my interest and goal. My strategic error was ultimately pointed out to me by Dr. Eliahu Caspi, a senior scientist at the Foundation, who taught me his simple adage: "Tell them what you have done so far." He explained that each paper should take no more than 2 weeks to complete. Taking his advice, I have never stopped writing since that day in 1974.

A New Strategy: Long-Term Adjuvant Tamoxifen

Upon my return to England in September 1974, my principal interest was to understand the pharmacology of tamoxifen and to devise a strategy for the best clinical application of an antiestrogen treatment. The drug had been available for the treatment of advanced breast cancer in Britain since 1973, but similar approval would not occur in the United States until 1978. Throughout this period, ICI Pharmaceuticals and the Yorkshire Cancer Research Campaign generously supported my laboratory at the University of Leeds in England. We devised the strategy of long-term (greater than 1 year) adjuvant tamoxifen therapy that was taken into clinical trials on both sides of the Atlantic. My group also discovered that a metabolite of tamoxifen, 4-hydroxytamoxifen, has a high affinity for the estrogen receptor but retains antiestrogenic activity. This set the stage for the subsequent discovery of numerous new antiestrogens that are currently being tested in clinical trials around the world.

ICI 46,474 had become tamoxifen. The scientific basis for prevention and long-term (greater than 1 year) adjuvant therapy had been established in the laboratory in 1977. These data would provide the rationale for the clinical development of antiestrogens for the next 20 years.

Chapter 1

Breast Cancer: Who and Why?

Monica Morrow, MD
Director, Lynn Sage Comprehensive
  Breast Program
Northwestern University Medical School

Breast cancer is the most common cancer in American women and the second most common cause of cancer death. Current estimates indicate that the lifetime risk of developing breast cancer is 12.2%, or 1 in 8 women, and the risk of breast cancer death is 3.6%, or 1 in 282.[1] The knowledge that breast cancer is a common disease, coupled with awareness on the part of both physicians and women of the factors that increase breast cancer risk, has caused concerns that breast cancer is an "epidemic," and has led many women to overestimate their level of risk.

Incidence

Everyone is familiar with the American Cancer Society statistic that 1 in 8 women will develop breast cancer. What many do not realize, however, is that this is a cumulative risk estimate, with half of a woman's risk occurring after the age of 65. As illustrated in Figure 1, age is a major breast cancer risk factor, with the majority of cancers occurring in women over age 55. The baseline risk for younger women, in the absence of other major risk factors, is quite low, and the chance of developing breast cancer between the ages of 35 and 55 is only 2.5 % (Table 1).[2] It is also noteworthy that these figures represent the risk of *developing* breast cancer, not the risk of *dying* from breast cancer. The risk of dying of the disease is substantially lower—only 3.6% in a woman's lifetime.

If these statistics are true, how can we explain the large number of breast cancer cases being seen today, particularly in younger women? An examination of breast cancer incidence (number of cases per 100,000 women) from 1970 to 1993 reveals a small but real increase in the incidence of the disease (Figure 2), which is evident for all age groups, but certainly does not qualify as an epidemic. What has changed dramatically during that time period, however, is the number of younger women at risk. As illustrated in Figure 3, the aging of the post-World War II baby boom generation has resulted in an increase in the absolute number of women at risk for breast cancer and a

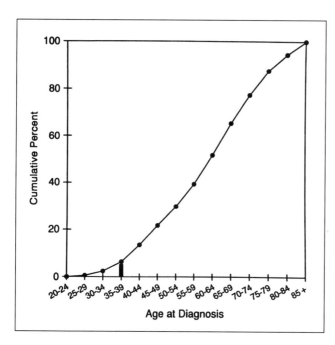

FIGURE 1 Cumulative distribution of breast cancer cases by age 1987-1989 Reprinted from Hankey BF et al: Monographs of the Journal of the National Cancer Institute 16:8, 1994.

corresponding increase in the absolute number of cases. Thus, in 1970, 5,120 cases of breast cancer in women under age 40 were reported to the SEER program. This increased to 7,800 cases in 1980 and 10,050 cases in 1990, while the actual incidence of the disease remained fairly stable.[1]

Risk Factors

As with many other cancers, the etiology of breast cancer appears to be multifactorial. Both endogenous and exogenous factors are known to increase breast cancer risk. In addition to age, family history, reproductive history, and benign breast disease are all endogenous factors that contribute to risk. Exposure to ionizing radiation is perhaps the most well documented exogenous risk factor, but diet, alcohol, pesticides, and electromagnetic fields have all been suggested to increase breast cancer risk. While most people recognize the existence of risk factors, the magnitude of the increase in risk associated with these factors is often poorly understood, and knowledge of the interactions among risk factors is limited.

Family History

Family history is probably the most widely recognized breast cancer risk factor. It is now apparent that there are two very different levels of risk in women with family histories of breast cancer, one due to a genetically inherited predisposition to breast cancer, and the other associated with an increased familial incidence of breast cancer. At present, mutations in three genes, p53, BRCA-1, and BRCA-2 have been associated with a genetic predisposition to breast cancer, and it is likely that additional genes will be identified in the future. Genetic breast cancer is uncommon, and is thought to account for only 5% to 10% of breast cancers in the US.[3,4] Familial characteristics suggestive of a genetic predisposition to breast cancer are listed in Table 2. The risk of genetic breast cancer associated with various combinations of these factors is shown in Table 3.

Since predisposing genes may be inherited from male or female relatives, and appear to be transmitted in an autosomal dominant fashion,[4] a breast cancer risk assessment should include an evaluation of both maternal and paternal family histories. In an individual woman with breast cancer, the possibility that the disease resulted from a predisposing gene is related to the age at which disease developed. It is estimated that 12% of women diagnosed with breast cancer before the age of 30 carry such a gene, compared with 3% diagnosed between ages 40 and 49.

BRCA-1

Mutations of the BRCA-1 gene, located on chromosome 17q21, are associated with a risk of both breast and ovarian cancer.[5] For women with these mutations, the risk of developing breast cancer before age 50 is estimated to be 50%, increasing to 85% by age 65. And, the risk of a second breast cancer is 65% by age 70.

The risk of ovarian cancer development is less well quantified and ranges

Table 1

Probability of Developing and Dying of Breast Cancer

Age (Years)	Risk of Breast Cancer Development	Risk of Breast Cancer Death
Birth-110	10.2%	3.6%
65-110	6.53%	1.53%
20-40	0.49%	0.09%
35-55	2.53%	0.56%
50-70	4.67%	1.04%
65-85	5.48%	1.01%

Data from Seidman et al.[2]

from 20% to 50%. Mutations of BRCA-1 also appear to be associated with a two-fold increase in the risk of prostate cancer, and a small increase in the risk of colon cancer. Recently, a specific mutation of BRCA-1 (185 delAG) was identified in 1% of a group of unrelated Ashkenazi Jewish women who had undergone testing for Tay Sachs disease.[6] This mutation may account for as many as 25% of breast cancer cases occurring in young Ashkenazi women, although further studies are needed to confirm this. To date, more than 100 different mutations of the BRCA-1 gene have been identified, and points out a major limitation in our knowledge of breast cancer genetics. As more women are tested, more and more mutations will be identified. The level of cancer risk associated with each of these individual mutations is uncertain, since estimates of risk established to date were derived from the study of a relatively small number of families selected for their very high incidence of breast cancer.

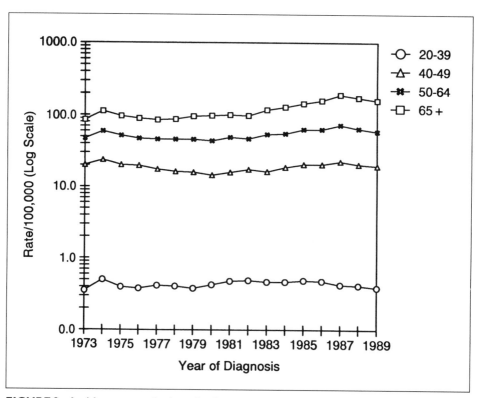

FIGURE 2   Incidence rates for invasive breast cancer 1979-1989, by age   Reprinted from Hankey BF et al: Monographs of the Journal of the National Cancer Institute 16:8, 1994.

Table 2

**Familial Characteristics Suggestive
of a Genetic Predisposition
to Breast Cancer**

Multiple relatives (usually > 3) with breast cancer

History of breast and ovarian cancer

Early onset breast cancer

Bilateral breast cancer

BRCA-2

Mutations of the BRCA-2 gene, located on chromosome 13, appear to carry the same level of breast cancer risk as mutations of BRCA-1.[7] With this genetic mutation, however, there is only a small increase in the risk of ovarian cancer. In addition, BRCA-2 mutations are associated with an increased risk of breast cancer in men.

In contrast to women with a genetic predisposition to breast cancer, women with an increased familial incidence of breast cancer have a much lower

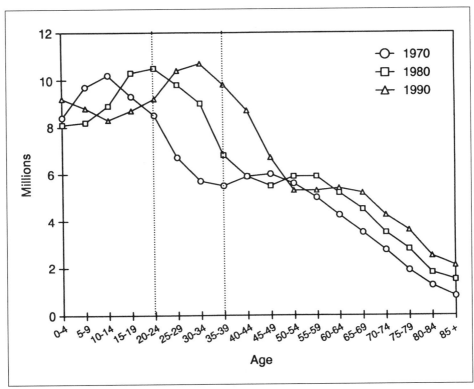

FIGURE 3 Changes in the age distribution of the US female population by year Reprinted from Hankey BF et al: Monographs of the Journal of the National Cancer Institute 15:9, 1994.

Table 3

Estimated Probability of Breast Cancer Being Due to the BRCA-1 Gene

Criterion, Cancer, Age (y)	Probability Case Has a BRCA-1 Mutation
Single Affected	
Breast < 30	0.12
Breast < 40	0.06
Breast 40 - 49	0.03
Ovarian < 50	0.07
Sister Pairs	
Breast < 40, Breast < 40	0.37
Breast 40 - 49, Breast 40-49	0.20
Breast < 50, Ovarian < 50	0.61
Families	
Breast only ≥ 3 cases, diagnosed < 50	0.40
≥ 2 breast, ≥ 1 ovarian	0.82
≥ 2 breast, ≥ 2 ovarian	0.91

risk of the disease. The level of risk in familial breast cancer varies according to the degree of closeness of the affected relative and the age at which the relative developed the disease.[8,9] As illustrated in Table 4, the cumulative risk of breast cancer development in a woman with familial breast cancer rarely exceeds 30%.

The preceding discussion makes it clear that the ability to identify carriers of breast cancer predisposition genes is of great value when counseling women about their personal levels of breast cancer risk. Nevertheless, there are a number of issues surrounding the practice of genetic testing that must be considered.

First, this is a technique that is in its infancy, and widespread standards for quality control have not yet been developed and false positive and false negative rates are unknown. Second, a positive test has the potential to produce severe anxiety, while a negative test may engender feelings of guilt, and either result can produce familial discord. In addition, genetic testing has the potential to reveal unsuspected information, such as the lack of a biologic

Table 4

Breast Cancer Risk in Familial, Nonhereditary Cases

Affected Relative, Age	% Risk by Age 80
One first degree, < 50	13%-21%
One first degree, > 50	9%-11%
One second degree, < 50	10%-14%
Two second degree, < 50	21%-26%
Two first degree, < 50	35%-48%
Two first degree, > 50	11%-24%

relationship with a parent. A positive test also carries enormous implications for insurability, so confidentiality is a major issue. Finally, a negative test does not necessarily eliminate the possibility of a genetic predisposition to breast cancer. For example, if a healthy woman with several affected relatives tests negative for a BRCA-1 mutation, it could mean that she does not carry the abnormal gene and is not at increased risk, or it could mean that BRCA-1 is not the gene responsible for breast cancer in her family. The information gained from testing will be greatly enhanced by testing a relative with breast cancer, as well as the non-affected woman who wants to know her genetic status.

The information presented above makes it clear that there are multiple uncertainties surrounding genetic testing. In addition, for the woman found to be at markedly elevated risk of breast cancer development, there are no satisfactory prevention strategies. For these reasons, some women at risk for genetic breast cancer may opt not to be tested for predisposition genes. Genetic testing is not simply the ordering of a blood test. A counselling session prior to a decision to be tested should include a discussion of the problems and uncertainties associated with testing. In women who opt to be tested, a follow-up session to discuss the meaning of test results and to develop a surveillance strategy is a necessity.

Hormonal Factors

Breast cancer is clearly related to hormones, and numerous studies have linked breast cancer incidence to the age of menarche, menopause, and first pregnancy. The greatest risk is associated with a long period of uninterrupted menstrual cycles. There appears to be a 20% decrease in breast cancer risk for each year that menarche is delayed,[10] and other factors that delay the establishment of regular ovulatory cycles, such as physical activity, may also decrease risk.[11] Age at menopause also influences breast cancer risk, with women whose natural menopause occurs before age 45 having half the relative risk of breast cancer of women whose menopause occurs after age

Table 5

Hormonal Risk Factors for Breast Cancer Development

Factor	Relative Risk
MENSTRUAL HISTORY	
Menarche < 12 yrs	1.3
Menopause > 55 yrs	1.5-2.0
Menopause < 45 yrs	0.77
PREGNANCY	
First live birth 25-29 yrs	1.5
First live birth after 30 yrs	1.9
First live birth after 35 yrs	2.0-3.0
Nulliparous	1.4-3.0

55.[12] Oophorectomy results in similar risk reductions.

Parity and age at first birth have also been shown to influence risk. Nulliparous women are at greater risk than those who are parous, with a relative risk of about 1.4. The effect of term pregnancy on risk varies with age at first birth, with women whose first pregnancy occurs after age 30 having a two- to five-fold increase in risk compared with women whose first term pregnancy is before age 18 or 19.[13,14] Abortion, whether spontaneous or induced, has no protective effect. Some studies have shown an increase in risk after incomplete pregnancy, while others show no effect. [15-17] The magnitude of increase in risk for hormonal risk factors is summarized in Table 5. Studies of the effect of lactation on breast cancer risk have had variable results, but recent studies have suggested that lactation for prolonged periods of time may reduce breast cancer risk in premenopausal women, while having little effect on the risk of postmenopausal breast cancer.[18,19]

The effect of exogenous hormones, in the form of oral contraceptives and hormone replacement therapy, has been extensively studied, but clear evidence of a major influence on risk is lacking. Overall, there is no convincing evidence of an increased risk of breast cancer in women who have ever used oral contraceptives.[20-22] Studies of women with family histories of breast cancer or of benign breast disease have also failed to demonstrate an increased risk when oral contraceptives are used.

Studies of hormone replacement therapy have produced more variable results, but two meta-analyses suggest small but statistically significant increases in risk (relative risk 1.3 and 1.06) related to the duration of estrogen use. [23,24] For the majority of women, however, the benefits of hormone replacement therapy in reducing the risk of cardiovascular disease and osteoporosis outweigh the small increase in breast cancer risk.

Dietary Factors

The observation that national per capita fat consumption is correlated with breast cancer incidence and mortality suggests a possible relationship between diet and breast cancer risk. Nevertheless, epidemiologic studies of fat consumption and breast cancer risk have been inconclusive. In the largest prospective study of dietary fat, 89,538 nurses between the ages of 34 and 59 were studied. No relationship between the intake of total fat, saturated fat, cholesterol, or linoleic acid and breast cancer risk was found.[25] A review of 10 prospective studies (Figure 4) also failed to demonstrate a relationship between dietary fat (within the context of Western diets) and risk.[26] However, these studies do not exclude the possibility that a low dietary fat intake in childhood or extremely low-fat diets may alter risk.

Evidence does exist which supports a relationship between alcohol intake and breast cancer risk. A meta-analysis of 12 case control studies demonstrated a relative risk of 1.4 for each 24 grams of alcohol consumed per day (about 2 drinks),[27] and data from prospective studies confirm this risk.[28,29] It is unclear, however, whether it is drinking early in life or ongoing drinking that increases risk.

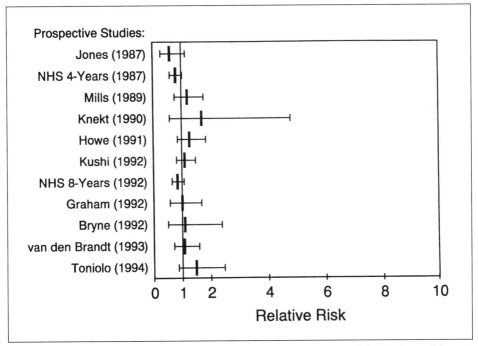

FIGURE 4 Prospective studies of the association between total fat intake and breast cancer Vertical bars represent the relative risk for the highest category of fat intake. Reprinted from Hunter D and Willet W: Dietary Factors in Diseases of the Breast. Lippincott-Raven p.203, 1996. With permission.

Benign Breast Disease

Benign breast lesions are classified as non-proliferative, proliferative, or atypical. Non-proliferative lesions are not associated with increased breast cancer risk and accounted for 69% of 10,000 biopsies reported by DuPont and Page.[30] Proliferative disease is associated with a small increase in breast cancer risk (relative risk, 1.5 to 2.0), while atypical hyperplasia carries the greatest risk of cancer development (relative risk 4-5).[30,31]

However, when strict diagnostic criteria are used, atypical hyperplasia is identified infrequently, and accounted for only 3.6% of the cases in the study of DuPont and Page. In this study, when atypical hyperplasia occurred in a woman with a family history of breast cancer, risk was substantially increased. The absolute risk of breast cancer development in women with a positive family history and atypical hyperplasia was 20% at 15 years, compared with 8% in women with atypical hyperplasia and a negative family history of breast cancer. Interestingly, no further increase in the risk of breast cancer was observed in women with proliferative disease who used estrogen after their breast biopsies.[32] The histologic diagnosis classified as proliferative, non-proliferative, and atypical are listed in Table 6.

Table 6

Classification of Benign Breast Disease

Nonproliferative: No Increase in Risk

Adenosis	Fibrosis
Cysts, Micro or Macro	Mastitis
Duct ectasia	Metaplasia, squamous or apocrine
Fibroadenoma	Mild hyperplasia

Proliferative: 1.5 to 2.0 Fold Increase in Risk

Moderate or florid hyperplasia

Sclerosing adenosis

Papilloma with fibrovascular core

Atypia: 4.0 to 5.0 Fold Increase in Risk

Atypical hyperplasia, lobular or ductal

Environmental Factors

Exposure to moderate to high dose ionizing radiation, either secondary to nuclear explosion or medical diagnostic and therapeutic procedures, increases breast cancer risk.[33-36] The level of risk is dependent on age at exposure, with a minimal increase in risk for exposure after age 40.[33-36] However, less than 1% of breast cancer is estimated to result from common radiologic diagnostic procedures such as chest x-rays or mammography.[37] Recently, a markedly increased risk of breast cancer development has been reported in women receiving mantle irradiation for the treatment of Hodgkin's disease

---

Table 7

History for Evaluation of Breast Cancer Risk

Patient Age

Reproductive History

Age of menarche

Parity, age at first birth

Age of menopause

Use of exogenous estrogen

Family History—Maternal and Paternal Relatives

Age at diagnosis, laterality of breast cancers

Presence of other cancer, especially ovarian

Number of unaffected relatives

Prior Biopsies

Number

Histologic diagnosis

Alcohol Intake

Exposure to Ionizing Radiation

---

before 15 years of age.[36] Other environmental factors, including exposure to electromagnetic fields, occupational exposures, and organochlorine pesticides, have been suggested to increase breast cancer risk,[38,39] but definitive data supporting these associations is lacking.

The High-Risk Woman

Although a number of factors which influence risk have been identified, there is no consensus as to what constitutes a "high-risk" woman. In addition, approximately 50% of women who develop breast cancer have no risk factors beyond being female and aging.[40] The designation of a woman as "high-risk" often results in unnecessary physician visits, frequent mammograms, and an excessive number of breast biopsies.

A risk evaluation begins with a careful history to evaluate the presence of known risk factors (Table 7) and a breast examination to exclude the presence of breast pathology and assess the difficulty of the examination. In women age 40 and older a mammogram should also be obtained. An attempt should then be made to provide the patient with a quantitative estimate of her absolute risk of breast cancer over a defined time interval, since most women overestimate the risk of developing the disease. A major problem in risk estimation has been the lack of knowledge of interactions among risk factors, since most studies have addressed only a single risk factor.

Gail et al[41] have developed a model that incorporates age at menarche, age at first live birth, number of first-degree relatives with breast cancer, and number of previous breast biopsies, to provide an individualized risk estimate for breast cancer development at different ages over various time intervals.

This model has been tested in the Texas Breast Screening Project and the Nurses Health Study populations and has been found to be generally accurate in women undergoing regular mammographic screening.[42,43] However, the model is not useful in estimating risk in women with strong family histories of breast cancer, since it includes only first-degree relatives.

At present, the options available to the high-risk woman are careful surveillance or prophylactic mastectomy.[44,45] The efficacy of careful surveillance, which usually consists of monthly breast self-examination, a physician breast examination every 4 to 6 months, and annual mammography, is unknown. Prophylactic mastectomy, although it clearly reduces breast cancer risk, is not 100% protective, and in this era of breast-conserving treatment for carcinoma is viewed by many as excessively radical. There are no absolute indications for prophylactic mastectomy, since the degree of breast cancer risk that is acceptable will vary among individuals. The long-term risk of breast cancer development in a population of high-risk women undergoing prophylactic mastectomy is uncertain.

Summary

Although a number of breast cancer risk factors have been identified, the mechanisms by which risk is increased remain uncertain, as do the interactions between factors that increase and decrease the risk of the disease. In addition, half of the women who develop breast cancer have no identifiable risk factors, indicating that strategies for the prevention and early detection of breast cancer must continue to be directed at the population of women as a whole to have an impact on breast cancer morbidity and mortality.

References

1. Miller BA, Feuer EJ, Hankey BF: The significance of the rising incidence of breast cancer in the United States. In: DeVita VT, Hellman S, Rosenberg SA (eds): *Important Advances in Oncology 1994.* p. 193. JB Lippincott, Phila, 1994.

2. Seidman H, Mushinski M, Gelb S: Probability of eventually developing or dying of breast cancer, United States. *CA Cancer J Clin* 35:36, 1985.

3. Claus E, Rich N, Thompson W. Genetic analysis of breast cancer in the Cancer and Steroid Hormone Study. *Am J Hum Genet* 48:232,1991.

4. Weber B, Garber J: Familial breast cancer. In: Harris J, Lippman M, Morrow M, Hellman S eds. Diseases of the Breast. Lippincott-Raven 1996:168.

5. Miki Y, Swensen J, Shattuck-Eidens D, et al: A strong candidate for the breast and ovarian cancer susceptibility gene BRCA-1. *Science* 266:66, 1994.

6. Strewing J, Abeliovich D, Peterz T, et al: The carrier frequency of the BRCA-1 185 delAG mutation is approximately 1 percent in Ashkenazi Jewish individuals. *Nat Genet* 11:198, 1995.

7. Wooster R, Neuhausen SL, Mangion J, et al: Localization of a breast cancer susceptibility gene, BRCA-2, to chromosome 13 q 12-13. *Science* 265:2088, 1994.

8. Hoskins KF, Stopfer JE, Calzone KA, et al: Assessment and counseling for women with a family history of breast cancer. A guide for clinicians. *JAMA* 273:577, 1995.

9. Claus EB, Risch NJ, Thompson WD: Autosomal dominant inheritance of early onset breast cancer. *Cancer* 73:643, 1994.

10. MacMahon B, Cole P, Brown J: Etiology of human breast cancer: A review. *J Natl Cancer Inst* 50:21, 1973.

11. Bernstein L, Ross R, Lobo R: The effects of moderate physical activity on menstrual cycle patterns in adolescence: Implications for breast cancer prevention. *Br J Cancer* 55:681, 1987.

12. Trichopoulos D, MacMahon B, Cole P: Menopause and breast cancer risk. *J Natl Cancer Inst* 48:605, 1972.

13. MacMahon B, Cole P, Lin T: Age at first birth and breast cancer risk. *Bull WHO* 43:209, 1970.

14. Trichopoulos D, Hsieh C, MacMahon B: Age at first birth and breast cancer risk. *Int J Cancer* 31:701, 1983.

15. Howe H, Senie R, Bzsuch H, et al: Early abortion and breast cancer risk in women under age 40. *Int J Epidemiol* 18:300, 1989.

16. Newcomb P, Storer B, Longnecker M, et al: Pregnancy termination in relation to risk of breast cancer. *JAMA* 275:283, 1996.

17. Adami H, Bergstrom R, Lund E et al. Absence of association between reproductive variables and the risk of breast cancer in young women in Sweden and Norway. *Br J Cancer* 62:122, 1990.

18. Newcomb P, Storer B, Longnecker M, et al. Lactation and a reduced risk of premenopausal breast cancer. *N Engl J Med* 330:81, 1994.

19. Yuan J, Yu M, Ross R, et al: Risk factors for breast cancer in Chinese women in Shanghai. *Cancer Res* 48:1949, 1988.

20. Romieu L, Berlin J, Colditz G: Oral contraceptives and breast cancer: Review and metaanalysis. *Cancer* 66:2253;1990.

21. Thomas D: Oral contraceptives and breast cancer: Review of the epidemiologic literature. *Contraception* 43:597 1991.

22. Malone K, Daling J, Weiss N: Oral contraceptives in relation to breast cancer. *Epidemiol Rev* 15:80, 1993.

23. Silleros-Arena M, Delgado-Rodriguez M, Rodigues-Canteras R, et al: Menopausal hormone replacement therapy and breast cancer: A metaanalysis. *Obstet Gynecol* 79:286;1992.

24. Steinberg K, Thacker S, Smith S, et al: A metaanalysis of the effect of estrogen replacement therapy on the risk of breast cancer. *JAMA.* 265:1985;1991.

25 Willett W, Stampfer M, Colditz G: Dietary fat and risk of breast cancer. *N Engl J Med* 316:22;1987.

26. Hunter DJ, Willett WC: Dietary factors in the etiology and pathogenesis of breast cancer. In Harris JR, Lippman ME, Morrow M, Hellman S (eds): *Diseases of the Breast* p. 201 Lippincott-Raven, 1996.

27. Longnecker M, Berlin J, Orza M, et al: A metaanalysis of alcohol consumption in relation to breast cancer risk. *JAMA.* 260:642;1988.

28. Gapstur S, Potter J, Sellers T, et al: Increased risk of breast cancer with alcohol consumption in postmenopausal women. *Am J Epidemiol* 136:1221, 1992.

29. Friedenreich C, Howe G, Miller A, et al: A cohort study of alcohol consumption and risk of breast cancer. *Am J Epidemiol* 137:512, 1993.

30. Dupont W, Page D: Risk factors for breast cancer in women with proliferative breast disease. *N Engl J Med* 312:146, 1985.

31. Hutter R: Consensus meeting: Is fibrocystic disease of the breast precancerous. *Arch Pathol Lab Med* 110:171, 1986.

32. Dupont W, Page D, Rogers L, et al: Influence of exogenous estrogens, proliferative breast disease, and other variables on breast cancer risk. *Cancer* 63:948, 1989.

33. Tokunaga M, Land C, Yamamoto T, et al: Incidence of female breast cancer among atomic bomb survivors, Hiroshima and Nagasaki. *Radiat Res* 112:243, 1987.

34. Miller A, Howe G, Sherman G: Mortality from breast cancer after irradiation during fluoroscopic examinations in patients being treated for tuberculosis. *N Engl J Med* 321:1285, 1989.

35. Hildreth N, Shore L, Dvorestsky P: The risk of breast cancer after irradiatio of the thymus in infancy. *N Engl J Med* 321:146, 1989.

36. Hancock S, Tucker M, Hoppe R: Breast cancer after treatment of Hodgkin's disease. *J Natl Cancer Inst* 85:25, 1993.

37. Evans JS, Wennberg JE, McNeil BJ: The influence of diagnostic radiography on the incidence of breast cancer and leukemia. *N Engl J Med* 315:819, 1986.

38. Loomis D, Savitz D, Ananth C: Breast cancer mortality among female electrical workers in the United States. *J Natl Cancer Inst* 86:921, 1994.

39. Wolff M, Toniolo P, Lee E, et al: Blood levels of organochlorine residues and risk of breast cancer. *J Natl Cancer Inst* 85:648, 1993.

40. Madigan M, Zeigler R, Benichon C, et al: Proportion of breast cancer cases in the United States explained by well established risk factors. *J Natl Cancer Inst* 87:1681, 1995.

41. Gail M, Brinton L, Byar D, et al: Projecting individualized probabilities of developing breast cancer for white females who are being examined annually. *J Natl Cancer Inst* 81:1879, 1989.

42. Bondy M, Lustbader E, Halabi S, et al: Validation of a breast cancer risk assessment model in women with a positive family history. *J Natl Cancer Inst* 86:620, 1994.

43. Spiegelman D, Colditz G, Hunter D, et al: Validation of the Gail et al model for predicting individual breast cancer risk. *J Natl Cancer Inst* 86:600, 1994.

44. Morrow M: Identification and management of the women at increased risk for breast cancer development. *Br Ca Res Treat* 31:53, 1994.

45. Bilimoria M, Morrow M: The woman at increased risk for breast cancer: Evaluation and management strategies. *CA Cancer J Clin* 45:263, 1995.

Chapter 2

Why Tamoxifen?

V. Craig Jordan, PhD, DSc
Director, Breast Cancer Research Program
Robert H. Lurie Cancer Center
Northwestern University Medical School

One hundred years ago, Dr. George Beatson[1] made the astonishing decision to treat advanced breast cancer in a premenopausal woman by removing her ovaries. Beatson was aware that farmers in Scotland could affect lactation in their animals by removal of the ovaries, so after completing preliminary studies in rabbits, he reasoned that the "ovarian irritation" of the mammary glands—breast cancer—in a woman might be influenced by the removal of her ovaries. Beatson initially reported that one of his patients had a dramatic response to the procedure, and by 1900 Stanley Boyd[2] at Charing Cross Hospital in London had collected the records of 46 premenopausal women (excluding 8 Edinburgh cases) with advanced breast cancer and documented their responses to oophorectomy. However, he observed that only one in three patients (actually 37%) responded to the procedure. The reason for this was to remain obscure for the next 60 years.

Estrogens: The Circulating Messengers of the Ovaries

What was remarkable about Beatson's original report in 1896 was that the endocrine role of the ovaries was completely unknown. In 1923, Drs. Allen and Doisy[3] in St. Louis described their finding of an "estrus stimulating principle" in the follicular fluid of pig ovaries. The ovaries were known to control reproductive functions and it was also known that female animals come into heat and accept males only at certain times in their reproductive cycles.

Allen and Doisy's studies illustrate the close relationship that is necessary between the laboratory and the clinic to unlock the mysteries of human physiology. They devised a test system for examining follicular fluid by first ovariectomizing mice and eliminating the reproductive cycle. They discovered that the vaginal epithelium undergoes the same cellular changes (called cornification) in response to injections of ovarian follicular fluid as the vagina does when the unovariectomized mouse goes into heat or "estrus" (from the

FIGURE I Professor Elwood V. Jensen He proposed the estrogen receptor system to explain responses to estrogens at estrogen target tissues and later devised the estrogen receptor assay to predict the hormonal dependency of breast cancer.

Latin word meaning *frenzy*). The chemicals produced by the ovaries that were subsequently identified as circulating messengers were named estrogens. It was thus discovered that these estrogens can selectively activate estrogen target tissues (uterus, vagina, breast) in a woman. The concept of endocrine control of one organ by a distant organ became an established fact.

Now we should return to the originial question regarding why some breast tumors respond to the removal of ovarian influence whereas others do not. In 1962, Drs. Elwood Jensen (Figure 1) and Herb Jacobson[4] synthesized radioactive estradiol, the most potent of the natural estrogens in a woman's body. With this breakthough, these investigators were able to address the question of differing tissue responses to estrogen. Although natural estrogens circulate throughout the female body, only target tissues become activated. Jensen and Jacobson injected radioactive estradiol into immature female rats (ie, animals that have no estrogen because their ovaries are inactive) and killed the animals at different times over the next 24 hours to find out where the estrogen had gone. They found that the radioactivity was initially bound to all tissues but was only retained in the estrogen target tissues (uterus and vagina). There must be a mechanism, they reasoned, a receptor that enabled the target tissues to retain estrogen.

The Estrogen Receptor Hypothesis

The estrogen receptor protein was subsequently isolated from the rat uterus in 1966 by parallel research ventures by Jensen's group at the University of Chicago and by Dr. Jack Gorski's group at the University of Illinois. The work rapidly translated to the clinic and established the concept of a pattern of estrogen target tissues containing the estrogen receptor through-

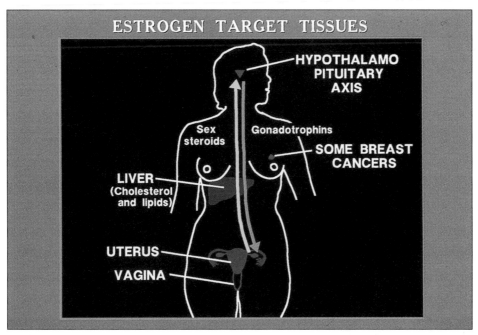

FIGURE 2   Sites commonly considered to be estrogen target tissues throughout a woman's body   Each site contains estrogen receptors within the cell to control the function of the tissue. The menstrual cycle is controlled through the hypothalamo-pituitary axis via feedback mechanisms that regulate ovarian steroidogenesis and ovulation. Similarly, estrogen regulates uterine biochemistry to prepare the tissue for progesterone action following ovulation in anticipation of successful ovum fertilization and implantation. Without implantation, steroidogenesis fails and menstruation occurs. Estrogen also controls circulating cholesterol through the regulation of liver metabolism, and estrogen maintains bone density (not shown). Some breast cancers contain the estrogen receptor and are considered to be estrogen target tissues.

out a woman's body (Figure 2).

Jensen's work, however, did not stop there. He reasoned that since estrogen controls estrogen action via the estrogen receptor, then perhaps breast cancer growth was regulated by the same mechanism. He established in the laboratory that some breast cancers did indeed contain the estrogen receptor, and he conducted the initial clinical studies illustrating the principle that patients whose tumor contains the estrogen receptor will respond to an endocrine maneuver, but those whose tumor was "estrogen receptor negative" were unlikely to respond.[5]

This principle was established in Bethesda, Maryland in 1974 at a National Cancer Institute-sponsored meeting. Investigators from around the world were invited to pool their clinical data on the usefulness of the estrogen-receptor assay to predict hormone responsive breast cancer. This conference was enormously successful and the consensus opinion revolutionized the treatment of breast cancer.[6] A patient with an estrogen-receptor-positive tumor has a 60% chance of responding to endocrine ablation, but a patient with an estrogen receptor-negative tumor has only a 10% chance of a response. Surgeons now had a test that could help them select women most likely to respond to endocrine ablation, and therefore reduce the cost and morbidity of treating everyone with ovarian or adrenal ablation. The test would avoid disappointing results in two thirds of patients.

Dramatic progress also was being made in a parallel research venture that would make endocrine ablation obsolete. There was a better way to treat patients—by blocking estrogen action in the tumor itself. If estrogen is the key that unlocks the growth mechanism in breast cancer, perhaps a drug that blocks the lock could be found and ablative surgery to remove the source of hormones could be avoided.

The First Antiestrogens

In 1958, Dr. Leonard Lerner[7] and co-workers at the William S. Merrell Company in Cincinnati reported their laboratory results with the first nonsteroidal antiestrogen, MER 25 or ethamoxytriphetol. The pharmacological properties of the drug were unique. Ethamoxytriphetol was antiestrogenic in every species tested[7] and the researchers could not detect any other hormonal or antihormonal activity. Theoretically, an antiestrogen could have many uses in gynecology or for the treatment of breast cancer. But it was the discovery that an antiestrogen could prevent pregnancy in laboratory animals—after they had mated—that seized the imagination of the pharmaceutical industry. Oral contraceptives were already established as effective agents to regulate fertility, but the tablets had to be taken daily throughout the cycle to suppress ovulation. Perhaps the antiestrogens would be effective "morning after pills" for occasional use?

Early clinical trials with ethamoxytriphetol demonstrated that the drug was active as an antiestrogen but had low potency and persistent troublesome side effects. These factors prevented further clinical evaluation. However, a successor compound, clomiphene, an analogue of the estrogen triphenylethylene (Figure 3), was found to be more potent than ethamoxytriphetol, and clinical trials were initiated.[8] Rather than acting as an antifertility agent, however, clomiphene appeared to actually induce ovulation, thus guaranteeing the precise effect it was supposed to prevent! To this day, clomiphene is used to induce ovulation in subfertile women.

ESTROGEN

Chlorotriphenylethylene

ANTIESTROGENS

Clomiphene
(mixture of <u>cis</u> and <u>trans</u> isomers)

Tamoxifen
(only the <u>trans</u> isomer)

FIGURE 3 Structural formula of triphenylethylene compounds (shown in bold) that have either estrogenic or antiestrogenic properties The key to antiestrogen activity is a correctly positioned alkyaminoethoxy side chain, illustrated by the two drugs in the lower part of the figure. Clomiphene is a mixture of two isomers with opposing biological properties. The *trans* isomer is an antiestrogen whereas the *cis* isomer is an estrogen. The diagram shows only the formula of the antiestrogenic *trans* isomer. The mixed isomers are used as an inducer of ovulation originally under the trade name Clomid. For comparison, the formula of tamoxifen is shown on the bottom right. It is the pure *trans* isomer only and is sold under the trade name of Nolvadex for the treatment of breast cancer.

Antiestrogens and Breast Cancer

During the 1960s, many pharmaceutical companies around the world were involved in the study of the structure activity relationships of the antiestrogens. Each compound was an effective antifertility agent in the laboratory rat, but it was clear that the property scientists were observing in animals did not translate into a clinically useful contraceptive. A number of preliminary clinical trials in breast cancer were conducted with several new antiestrogens because of the recognized link between estrogen and the growth of some breast cancers. It had also been found in the laboratory that antiestrogens could block the binding of radioactive estradiol in its target tissues, so the rationale for clinical studies in the 1970s was strong.

The Upjohn company in Kalamazoo, Michigan conducted extensive tests on their new antiestrogen, nafoxidine, but in the 1970s, after numerous clinical studies around the world, development was abandoned because all patients suffered severe toxic side effects.[9] Similarly clomiphene, an impure mixture of geometric isomers, was tested but concerns about potential toxicities, particularly cataracts, prevented further clinical development for long-term treatment. Clinical studies were abandoned in the early 1970s.[8]

ICI 46,474 to Tamoxifen

Scientists in the fertility control program of the pharmaceuticals division of Imperial Chemical Industries (ICI) in England were particularly interested in the discovery of the new nonsteroidal antiestrogens. The most potent nonsteroidal estrogen, diethylstilbestrol, had been discovered by Sir Charles Dodds in the late 1930s; structural analogs, the triphenylethylenes (Figure 3), were subsequently found to be potent, long-acting estrogenic drugs. ICI had already provided the triphenylethylenes to Sir Alexander Haddow for his pioneering studies[10]

FIGURE 4 Dr. Dora Richardson Co-patent holder for ICI46,474 and the organic chemist responsible for the synthesis of triphenylethylenes at ICI Pharmaceuticals, Macclesfield, Cheshire, England. This photograph was taken on the occasion of her retirement in 1979.

on the value of high-dose estrogen therapy to treat advanced breast cancer in postmenopausal women and to treat prostate cancer in men. This breakthrough in 1944 established a somewhat paradoxical, but effective, therapeutic option that is used today.

What interested the scientists at ICI was the fact that the new antiestrogens were derivatives of the estrogen triphenylene (Figure 3), but it was clear that improvements in the toxicity profiles and potencies had to be made before any clinically useful agent could be developed for long-term therapy.

Dr. Dora Richardson (Figure 4) began the process by systematically synthesizing numerous analogs of triphenylethylene. The breakthrough came in the mid-1960s when Drs. Harper and Walpole discovered that the *trans* isomer of a triphenylethylene, ICI 46,474, was the antiestrogenic compound of choice, whereas its *cis* geometric isomer ICI 47,699 was an estrogen in all tests.[11] Although the option as a fertility regulator was kept open—in fact, tamoxifen, as it became known, was marketed during the 1970s in Great Britain and Ireland for the induction of ovulation—Walpole suggested using tamoxifen as a treatment for breast cancer. Earlier in his career, Walpole had established a solid reputation as a cancer researcher, and he had conducted clinical studies with triphenylethylenes in the treatment of breast cancer in the 1940s.[12] ICI 46,474 had antiestrogenic activity in rats and primates, but would it work as an antitumor agent in women with breast cancer?

Table 1

Comparison of Early Clinical Experience with Antiestrogens as a Treatment for Advanced Breast Cancer

Antiestrogen	Daily Dose	Year	Response Rate	Toxicity
Ethamoxytriphetol	500-4500 mg	1960	25%	acute psychotic episodes
Clomiphene	100-300 mg	1964-1974	34%	fear of cataracts
Nafoxidine	180-240 mg	1976	31%	cataracts, ichthyosis, photophobia
Tamoxifen	20-40 mg	1971-1973	31%	transient thrombocytopenia*

*"The particular advantage of this drug is the low incidence of troublesome side effects." Cole et al: *Br J Cancer* 25:270-275, 1971.

"Side effects were usually trivial." Ward: *Br Med J* 1:13-14, 1973.

Dr. Mary Cole and co-workers at the Christie Hospital in Manchester, England, conducted the first preliminary evaluation of ICI 46, 474 for the palliative treatment of breast cancer. Initially, 46 postmenopausal patients with late-stage disease were treated with the drug; 10 patients responded. These results were subsequently confirmed in a small dose-response study by Dr. Harold Ward in Birmingham, England.

Tamoxifen Goes Forward Alone

The late Dr. Arthur Walpole deserves the credit for pursuing the application of tamoxifen as a potential palliative treatment for advanced breast cancer in postmenopausal women.[12] Tamoxifen, however, was only one of numerous compounds being tested by pharmaceutical companies during the 1960s. Table 1 compares and contrasts the different compounds that underwent evaluation. ICI Pharmaceuticals Ltd. (Zeneca) had the good fortune to discover a potent antiestrogen with a low profile of toxic side effects.

It was clear at the outset that tamoxifen had several advantages compared to the other contenders. Tamoxifen had higher antitumor potency (ie, a lower dose could be used) compared with other compounds being evaluated at the time. Moreover, while side effects represented a major problem with the other antiestrogens, tamoxifen had virtually no side effects. In fact, tamoxifen seemed to have none of the troublesome side effects observed with high-dose estrogen therapy or androgen therapy that were standard treatments at the time. Based on experience with drugs such as clomiphene, investigators were also concerned about the potential for long-term therapy to lead to cataract development. Even during the 1960s, however, the Zeneca scientists believed that tamoxifen would not produce cataracts. This has proved to be true after 20 years of use.

Back in the 1960s and '70s, Zeneca was the only company that had chosen to develop an antiestrogenic drug for the treatment of advanced breast cancer. However, there was little enthusiasm from the clinical community about this innovation—all hopes seemed pinned instead on the discovery and application of new cytotoxic chemotherapeutic agents. Clinical researchers 25 years ago reasoned that their only hope of curing breast cancer lay in the development of better and stronger cytotoxics. That perspective would eventually change when tamoxifen was successfully developed as a treatment for all stages of breast cancer .

References

1.   Beatson GT: On the treatment of inoperable cases of carcinoma of the mamma: Suggestions for a new method of treatment with illustrative cases. *Lancet* 2:104-107, 1896.

2. Boyd S: On oophorectomy in cancer of the breast. *Br Med J* 2:1161-1167, 1900.

3. Allen E, Doisy EA: An ovarian hormone: Preliminary report on its localisation, extraction, and partial purification and action in test animals. *JAMA* 81:819-821, 1923.

4. Jensen EV, Jacobson HI: Basic guides to the mechanism of estrogen action. *Recent Prog Horm Res* 18:387-414, 1962.

5. Jensen EV, Block GE, Smith S, et al: Estrogen receptors and breast cancer response to adrenalectomy, in Hall TC (ed): Prediction of response in cancer therapy. *Monogr Natl Cancer Inst* 34:55-70, 1971.

6. McGuire WL, Carbone PP, Vollmer EP (eds): *Estrogen Receptors in Human Breast Cancer.* New York, Raven Press, 1975.

7. Lerner LJ, Holthaus FJ, Thompson CR: A nonsteroidal estrogen antagonist 1-p-2 diethylaminoethoxyphenyl -1- phenyl 2-p- methoxyphenyethanol. *Endocrinology* 63:215-318, 1958.

8. Lerner LJ, Jordan VC: Development of antiestrogens and their use in breast cancer: Eighth Cain Memorial Award Lecture. *Cancer Res* 50:4177-4189, 1990.

9. Jordan VC: Origins of antiestrogens, in Lindsey R, Dempster D, Jordan VC (eds): *Estrogens and Antiestrogens,* Philadelphia, Lippincott, Raven (in press).

10. Haddow A, Wakinson JN, Patterson E, et al: Influence of synthethic oestrogens upon malignant disease. *Br Med J* 2:4368-4371, 1944.

11. Harper MJK, Walpole AL: A new deriative of triphenylethylene: Effect on implantation and mode of action in rats. *J Reprod Fertil* 13:101-117, 1967.

12. Jordan VC: The development of tamoxifen for breast cancer therapy: A tribute to the late Arthur Walpole. *Breast Cancer Res Treat* 11:197-209, 1988.

Chapter 3

The Clinical Development of Tamoxifen

V. Craig Jordan, PhD, DSc

In 1973, Nolvadex, the ICI brand of tamoxifen (as its citrate salt), was approved by the Committee on the Safety of Medicines in the United Kingdom for the treatment of breast cancer. Similarly, approval was given in the United States for the treatment of advanced disease in postmenopausal women by the Food and Drug Administration on December 30, 1977. Nolvadex is now available in more than 110 countries as first-line endocrine therapy for the treatment of breast cancer. To mark this achievement, ICI Ltd. Pharmaceuticals Division (Zeneca) was presented with the Queen's Award for Technological Achievement by the Lord Lieutenant of Cheshire, Viscount Leverhulme, on July 6, 1978 (Figures 1 and 2). The remarkable success of tamoxifen encouraged a closer examination of its pharmacology with a view to further development and wider applications.

Tamoxifen Metabolism

The metabolism of tamoxifen in animals and patients was first described by Fromson and co-workers at Zeneca. The major metabolic route to be described was hydroxylation to form 4-hydroxytamoxifen, which was subsequently shown to have high binding affinity for the estrogen receptor and be a potent antiestrogen in its own right, with antitumor properties in the DMBA model. Indeed, it is an advantage for tamoxifen to be metabolically activated to 4-hydroxytamoxifen, but this is not a prerequisite for antiestrogen action. The metabolite was subsequently shown to localize in target tissues after the administration of radioactive tamoxifen to rats.

Originally, 4-hydroxytamoxifen was believed to be the major metabolite of tamoxifen in patients, but Hugh Adam at Zeneca demonstrated that N-desmethyltamoxifen is the principal metabolite found in patients (Figure 3). There is usually a blood-level ratio of 2:1 for N-desmethyltamoxifen to tamoxifen in patients maintained on tamoxifen therapy, since N-desmethyltamoxifen has twice the plasma half-life of tamoxifen (14 days vs 7 days).

The ubiquitous use of tamoxifen in recent years has resulted in the publication of numerous methods to estimate tamoxifen and its metabolites in

FIGURE 1 **Celebrations at ICI pharmaceuticals division on the occasion of the presentation of the Queen's Award for Technological Achievement** At the head table are seated (left to right) Dr. Barry Furr, Deputy Chairman Alan Hayes, Dr. Dora Richardson, Viscount Leverhulm, Division Chairman Peter Cunliff, and the Mayor of Macclesfield.

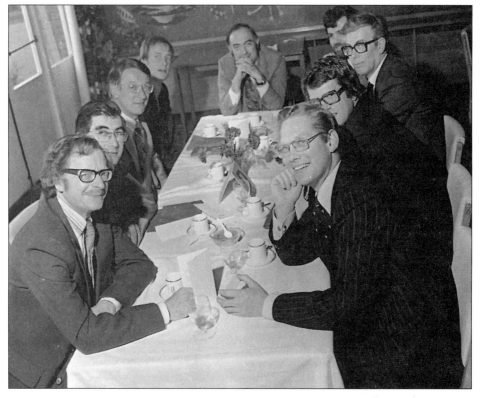

FIGURE 2 **Clinical development team for tamoxifen present at the presentation of the Queen's Award for Technological Achievement** Front left, Dr. Roy Cotton, who was initially in charge of clinical development; front right, the author, and behind, Dr. Sandy Todd.

serum.[1] The metabolites that have been identified in patients are shown in Figure 4. The minor metabolites—metabolite-Y, metabolite-Z, and 4-hydroxy-N-desmethyltamoxifen—may all contribute to the antitumor actions of tamoxifen because they are all antiestrogens which inhibit the binding of estradiol to the estrogen receptor.

Blocking Growth of Breast Cancer Cells

The next significant advance in the understanding of tamoxifen action in breast cancer came with the availability of hormone-dependent human breast cancer to study anti-tumor mechanisms in the laboratory. In 1975, Marc

FIGURE 3 Original metabolites of tamoxifen found in human serum Although N-desmethyltamoxifen is the major metabolite and is present at about twice the concentration of tamoxifen in patient's serum, the minor metabolite 4-hydroxytamoxifen, has a high-binding affinity for the estrogen receptor and may contribute significantly to antitumor effects.

FIGURE 4 Metabolites of tamoxifen found in humans

Lippman[2] at the National Cancer Institute was the first to describe the ability of tamoxifen to inhibit the growth of MCF-7 estrogen-receptor-positive breast cancer cells in culture and to demonstrate that the addition of estrogen could reverse the action of tamoxifen. Nearly a decade later, Kent Osborne[3] in San Antonio and Rob Sutherland[4] in Australia independently described the blockade by tamoxifen of breast cancer cells at the G1 phase of the cell cycle.

Adjuvant Tamoxifen: Laboratory Studies to Clinical Trials

Throughout the 1970s and '80s, the development of tamoxifen became a conversation between the laboratory and the clinic (see Figure 5). The initial

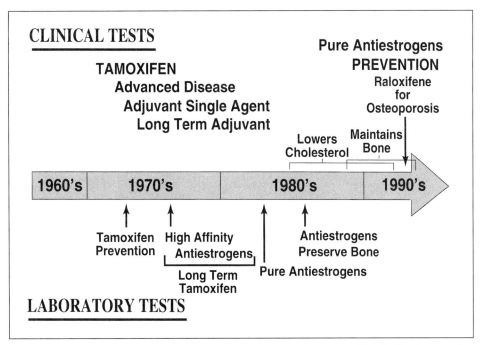

FIGURE 5 Laboratory and clinical development of tamoxifen The finding in 1973 that tamoxifen could prevent mammary cancer in rats ultimately led to breast cancer prevention trials in the 1990s. The 1977 laboratory finding that long-term treatment was superior to short-term treatment led to longer-than-1-year tamoxifen arms in adjuvant clinical trials. The discovery in 1976 of compounds with a high affinity for the estrogen receptor led to the development of new compounds like raloxifene that are being tested in clinical trials as a preventive for osteoporosis. Although it appears to be paradoxical that an "antiestrogen" could maintain rather than decrease bone density, the principle was first illustrated in the laboratory in 1987. It was tested with tamoxifen in clinical trials in postmenopausal women in the late 1980s, and subsequently used as justification for the development of raloxifene as a new targeted antiestrogen or selective estrogen receptor modulator (SERM).

success of adjuvant monotherapy with L-phenylalanine mustard or combination chemotherapy in the mid-1970s to delay the recurrence of node-positive breast cancer helped to encourage the investigation of other, perhaps less toxic therapies. Laboratory studies using the DMBA-induced rat mammary carcinoma model were first used to explore whether tamoxifen would be effective and whether the drug produced a tumoristatic or tumoricidal effect in vivo.

Studies in vitro by Marc Lippman had previously indicated that tamoxifen could be a tumoricidal drug, but the results from the in vivo DMBA studies (first reported at a breast cancer symposium at King's College, Cambridge, England in September 1977—Figure 6) demonstrated that a 1-month course of tamoxifen therapy given 1 month after the carcinogenic insult only delayed the appearance of mammary tumors; continuous therapy for 6 months, on the other hand, resulted in 90% of the animals remaining tumor-free (Figure 7). Indeed, tumors appeared whenever tamoxifen therapy was stopped.[5] Thus, tamoxifen was shown to have a tumoristatic component to its mode of action and the laboratory results indicated that long-term (up to 5 years) or indefinite therapy might be the best clinical strategy for adjuvant tamoxifen treatment.[6,7]

Subsequent laboratory studies using DMBA or N-nitrosomethylurea (NMU)-induced rat mammary tumors or human breast cancer cell lines inoculated into athymic mice have all supported that initial observation. However, attention now focussed on the clinical evaluation of the laboratory concept.

Several trials of tamoxifen monotherapy as an adjuvant to mastectomy were initiated in the mid- to late-1970s. The majority of clinical trials organizations selected a conservative course of 1 year of adjuvant tamoxifen therapy.

FIGURE 6 (right)   Participants at a Breast Cancer Symposium in September 1977 at Kings College, Cambridge, England   The concept of extended adjuvant tamoxifen treatment was first proposed at this meeting. Clinical studies of 1-year adjuvant tamoxifen were in place; regrettably, a decade later, this approach was shown to produce little survival benefit for patients. In the insets, (top) the author, who presented the new concept; (bottom left) Professor Michael Baum, the session chairman, who was about to launch the Nolvadex Adjuvant Trial Organization (NATO) 2-year adjuvant tamoxifen trial; and (bottom right) Dr. Helen Stewart, who was a participant at the conference. She would initiate a pilot trial in 1978 and, led by Sir Patrick Forest, would later guide the full randomized Scottish Trial of 5 years adjuvant tamoxifen treatment vs control in the 1980s. Both clinical trials were later proven to produce survival advantages for patients. The concept of longer tamoxifen treatment producing more survival benefits for patients was eventually established indirectly by the Oxford Overview Analysis in 1989 and directly by the Stockholm group led by Dr. Lars Rutqvist (Proc. ASCO 1996. Abstract 171 page 126).

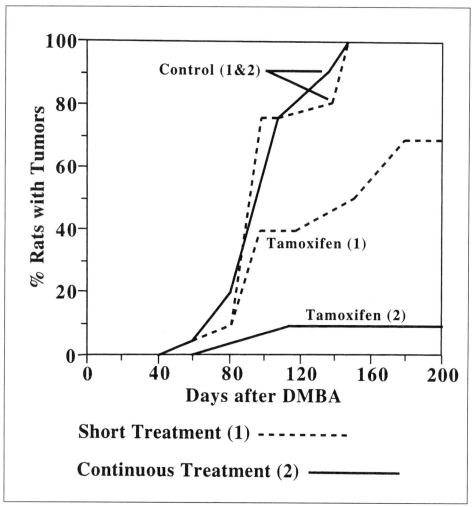

FIGURE 7   **The effectiveness of long-term tamoxifen treatment in the dimethylbenzan-thracene (DMBA)-induced rat mammary carcinoma model**   The administration of 20 mg DMBA by gavage to 50-day-old female Sprague Dawley rats results in all animals developing mammary tumors 160 days later. The short-term (30 days) administration of different daily doses (12.5-800 µg) of tamoxifen between days 30 and 60 after DMBA results in a delay in tumor formation. However, not all animals are protected from the carcinogen. In contrast, the daily administration of a clinically relevant dose (50 µg daily = 0.25 mg/kg in rats or 20 mg daily to a 70 kg woman) of tamoxifen continuously, starting 30 days after DMBA results in 90% of animals remaining tumor free.

This decision was based on a number of reasonable concerns. Patients with advanced disease usually respond to tamoxifen for 1 year, and it was expected that ER-negative disease would be encouraged to grow prematurely during adjuvant therapy. If this growth occurred, then the physician would have already used a valuable palliative drug and would have only combination chemotherapy to slow the relentless growth of recurrent disease. A related argument involved the changing strategy for the application of adjuvant combination chemotherapy. Recurrent treatment cycles (2 years) were found to be of no long-term benefit for patients. In contrast, it seemed that aggressive, short-term courses of treatment (6 months) with the most active cytotoxic drugs had the best chance to kill tumor cells before the premature development of drug resistance. The same intuitive sense that "longer might not be better" contributed to a reluctance on the part of the researchers to start with long-term tamoxifen therapy.

The remarkable success of tamoxifen encouraged a closer examination of its pharmacology

Finally, there were sincere concerns about the side effects of adjuvant therapy and the ethical issues of treating patients who might never have recurrent disease. Although this argument primarily focused on chemotherapy and node-negative patients, it is fair to say that few women in the mid-1970s had received extended therapy with tamoxifen—so that long-term side effects were largely unknown. Most tamoxifen-treated patients had only received about 2 years of treatment for advanced disease before drug resistance developed. Potential side effects, such as thrombosis and osteoporosis, were only of secondary importance. The use of tamoxifen in the disease-free patient, however, would change that perspective.

In 1977, Dr. Douglas C. Tormey and I organized the first evaluation of long-term tamoxifen therapy in node-positive patients treated with combination chemotherapy plus tamoxifen.[8] This pilot study was initiated to determine whether patients could tolerate 5 years of adjuvant tamoxifen therapy and whether metabolic tolerance would occur during long-term treatment. No unusual side effects of tamoxifen therapy were noted, and blood levels of tamoxifen and its metabolites N-desmethyltamoxifen and metabolite-Y remained stable throughout the 5 years of treatment. Although this study was not a randomized trial, those patients who received long-term tamoxifen therapy continued to make excellent progress, and many patients have been taking the drug for more than 14 years now. We have recently reported that tamoxifen does not produce metabolic tolerance during 10 years of administration. Serum levels of tamoxifen and its metabolites are maintained.[9]

Randomized Trials

These data and the DMBA rat mammary carcinoma data were used to support randomized ECOG trials EST 4181 and 5181. An early analysis of EST 4181, which compares short-term tamoxifen with long-term tamoxifen (both with combination chemotherapy), has demonstrated an increase in disease-free survival with long-term tamoxifen therapy. In fact, the 5-year tamoxifen arm has now gone through a second randomization, either to stop the tamoxifen or to continue the antiestrogen indefinitely.

Building on the success of these earlier trials that demonstrated the efficacy of tamoxifen in receptor-positive postmenopausal patients, the National Surgical Adjuvant Breast and Bowel Project (NSABP) has conducted a 2-year registration study of combination chemotherapy (L-PAM, 5FU) plus tamoxifen, with an additional year of tamoxifen alone. Overall, these investigators concluded that 3 years of tamoxifen confers a significant advantage over 2 years of tamoxifen.

A recent report from Italy has demonstrated that the addition of combination chemotherapy (CMF for six cycles followed by five courses of epirubicin) to long-term tamoxifen (5 years) therapy does not seem to improve significantly the clear-cut effectiveness of tamoxifen alone to prevent recurrence in ER- and node-positive disease.[10]

While the 2-year adjuvant tamoxifen study that was conducted by the Nolvadex Adjuvant Trials Organization or "NATO" (an acronym chosen to encourage American investigators to read Lancet papers because they might believe the work had been done by the North Atlantic Treaty Organization!)[11] was the first to demonstrate a survival advantage, current clinical trials are all evaluating a longer duration of tamoxifen therapy. A small, randomized clinical trial conducted in France has demonstrated a survival advantage for estrogen-receptor-positive patients who received 3 years of tamoxifen versus no treatment. Similarly, a Scottish trial (*The Lancet*, July 25, 1987) that evaluated 5 years of tamoxifen vs no treatment demonstrated a survival advantage for patients who take tamoxifen.[12] The Scottish trial is particularly interesting because it addresses the question of whether to administer tamoxifen early as an adjuvant or to save the drug until disease recurs. This comparison was possible because most patients in the control arm received tamoxifen at recurrence. Early concerns that long-term adjuvant tamoxifen would result in premature drug resistance are unjustified, since patients on the adjuvant tamoxifen arm had a survival advantage.

Conclusion

During the past 20 years, tamoxifen has moved from the laboratory to become the endocrine treatment of choice for all stages of breast cancer. The drug has a remarkable profile of interesting pharmacological effects: on one hand, tamoxifen can inhibit estrogen-stimulated breast cancer growth, while on the other hand, it can mimic some of the physiological functions of estrogen to support bone and lower circulating cholesterol.

The following chapters in this volume are intended to provide an up-to-date appraisal of the effectiveness and side effects of long-term tamoxifen therapy. For the future, the clinical trials that are testing the worth of tamoxifen as a preventive for breast cancer in normal women will provide the physician with a new therapeutic dimension that, it is hoped, will contribute to the improved health of thousands of women.

References

1. Langen-Fahey SM, Jordan VC, Fritz NF, et al: Clinical pharmacology and endocrinology of long-term tamoxifen therapy, in Jordan VC (ed): *Long Term Tamoxifen Treatment for Breast Cancer* pp 27-56, Madison, University of Wisconsin Press, 1994.

2. Lippman ME, Bolan G: Oestrogen responsive human breast cancer in long-term tissue culture. *Nature* 256:592-593, 1975.

3. Osborne CK, Boldt DH, Clark GH, et al: Effects of tamoxifen on human breast cancer cell cycle kinetics accumulation of cells in early G1 phase. *Cancer* 43:3583-3585, 1993.

4. Sutherland RL, Reddel RR, Green MD: Effects of oestrogens on cell proliferation and cell cycle kinetics: A hypothesis on the cell cycle effects of antiestrogens. *Eur J Cancer Clin Oncol* 19:307-318, 1983.

5. Jordan VC: Use of the DMBA-induced rat mammary carcinoma system for the evaluation of tamoxifen as a potential adjuvant therapy: Reviews on *Endoc Rel Cancer* (October Suppl) 49-55, 1978.

6. Jordan VC, Dix CJ, Allen KE: The effectiveness of long-term treatment in laboratory model for adjuvant hormone therapy of breast cancer, in Salmon SE, Jones SE (ed): *Adjuvant Therapy of Cancer* pp 19-24, New York, Grune and Stratton, 1979.

7. Jordan VC: Laboratory studies to develop general principles for the adjuvant treatment of breast cancer with antiestrogens: Problem and potential for future clinical applications. *Breast Cancer Res Treat* 3(Suppl):73-86, 1983.

8. Tormey DC, Jordan VC: Long-term tamoxifen adjuvant therapy in node positive breast cancer: A metabolic and pilot clinical study. *Breast Cancer Res Treat* 4:297-302, 1984.

9. Langan-Fahey SM, Tormey DC, Jordan VC: Tamoxifen metabolites in patients on long-term therapy for breast cancer. *Eur J Cancer* 26:883-888, 1990.

10. Boccardo F, Amorosso D, Rubagotti A, et al: Prolonged tamoxifen treatment of early breast cancer: The experience of the Italian Co-operative group for chemohormonal

therapy of early breast cancer, in Jordan VC (ed): *Long-Term Tamoxifen Treatment for Breast Cancer* pp 159-179, Madison, University of Wisconsin Press, 1994.

11. Nolvadex Adjuvant Trial Organization: Controlled trial of tamoxifen as a single adjuvant agent in the management of early breast cancer: Interim analysis at four years. *Lancet* i:257-261, 1983.

12. Breast Cancer Trials Committee, Scottish Cancer Trials Office (MRC): Adjuvant tamoxifen in the management of operable breast cancer: The Scottish Trial. *Lancet* ii:171-175, 1987.

Chapter 4

Current Approved Uses of Tamoxifen and Recommendations in the United States

V. Craig Jordan, PhD, DSc

Medicines are approved for use in the United States by the Food and Drug Administration (FDA). Approval for use in humans is made initially after a vigorous evaluation of preclinical, clinical, and toxicologic data by expert committees. Formal approval for use is made following the public deliberations of the expert committee which at that time recommends approval or disapproval of a product. Without approval of a medicine, the product cannot be marketed in the US and without approval of an indication, a company cannot promote the use of their product for that application.

Tamoxifen (Nolvadex) has been approved by the FDA for the treatment of advanced breast cancer in postmenopausal women since 1977. The product has been marketed in the US since then, and similar approvals have been obtained in 110 other countries. Tamoxifen has been used by millions of women worldwide and is currently the most frequently prescribed cancer drug.

During the past 20 years, additional approvals have been obtained from the FDA for other applications of tamoxifen. In 1985 tamoxifen was approved as an adjuvant therapy with chemotherapy in postmenopausal women with node-positive breast cancer, and in 1986 approval was obtained for the use of adjuvant tamoxifen alone in the same group of postmenopausal women with node-positive breast cancer.

In 1989, approval was obtained from the FDA for the use of tamoxifen in the treatment of premenopausal women with estrogen receptor-positive advanced breast cancer, and in 1990, an indication as an adjuvant was approved for pre- and postmenopausal patients with node-negative, estrogen-receptor-positive breast cancer.

Tamoxifen is also active in the treatment of male breast cancer, and in 1993 the FDA approved the use of tamoxifen to treat advanced breast cancer in men.

Table I

Adjuvant Treatment for Patients with Lymph-Node-Negative Breast Cancer*

Patient Group	Minimal-Low Risk	Good Risk	High Risk
PREMENOPAUSAL			
ER-positive	No adjuvant treatment vs tamoxifen†	**Tamoxifen** Oophorectomy† Chemotherapy† Gonadotropin-releasing hormone analogue†	**Chemotherapy** ± tamoxifen† Oophorectomy† Gonadotropin-releasing hormone analogue†
ER-negative	Not applicable	Not applicable	**Chemotherapy**
POSTMENOPAUSAL			
ER-positive	No adjuvant treatment versus tamoxifen†	**Tamoxifen**	**Tamoxifen** ± chemotherapy†
ER-negative	Not applicable	Not applicable	**Chemotherapy** ± tamoxifen†
ELDERLY	No adjuvant treatment versus tamoxifen†	**Tamoxifen**	**Tamoxifen;** if ER negative: **chemotherapy** ± tamoxifen†

*Bold entries are treatments accepted for routine use or baseline in clinical trials.

†Treatments still being tested in randomized clinical trials.

ER = estrogen receptor.

From Goldhirsch, Wood, Senn, et al: *J Natl Cancer Inst* 87:1441-1445, 1995.

Table 2

Adjuvant Treatment for Patients
with Lymph-Node-Positive Breast Cancer*

Patient Group	Treatment
PREMENOPAUSAL	
ER-positive	**Chemotherapy** ± tamoxifen†
	Ovarian ablation ± tamoxifen†
	Gonadotropin-releasing hormone analogue†
	Chemotherapy ± ovarian ablation (gonadotropin releasing hormone analogue) ± tamoxifen†
ER-negative	**Chemotherapy**
POSTMENOPAUSAL	
ER-positive	**Tamoxifen** ± chemotherapy
ER-negative	**Chemotherapy** ± tamoxifen†
ELDERLY	**Tamoxifen**; if ER negative: **chemotherapy** ± tamoxifen†

*Bold entries are treatments accepted for routine use or baseline in clinical trials.
†Treatments still being tested in randomized trials.
ER = estrogen receptor.
From Goldhirsch, Wood, Senn et al: *J Natl Cancer Inst* 87:1441-1445, 1995.

Overall, tamoxifen has repeatedly been shown to increase the survival of patients with breast cancer. Therefore, in 1994 the FDA approved the claim that tamoxifen prolonged the overall survival of the breast cancer patient.

The role of the FDA is to protect the general public from excessive claims of manufacturers of medicines. The system provides strict control of manufacturers and what can be claimed in their advertising to physicians. The aim is to ensure that physicians are not misled into believing false claims for a medicine.

Outside the relationship between physicians and pharmaceutical advertising, a physician has the authority to prescribe medicines that he or she believes will aid the patient; physicians can also use medicines in the context of an approved clinical trial. In the latter case, the patient is expected to read and sign an informed consent form stating the potential benefits and side effects of the experimental approach. Clinical trials are strictly controlled and monitored to safeguard the patient. No clinical trial provides less than the accepted standards of care.

Periodically, physicians meet to provide guidelines for the profession about the suggested treatment approaches for patients with breast cancer. These are called consensus conferences. The conclusions of the St. Gallen (Switzerland) breast cancer conference, for example, are published periodically in the Journal of the National Cancer Institute. The recommendations offered in 1995 by the international clinical community are summarized in the two tables: adjuvant treatment for patients with lymph-node-negative breast cancer (Table 1) and lymph-node-positive breast cancer (Table 2).

Chapter 5

Overviews of Adjuvant Tamoxifen Therapy

I. Craig Henderson, MD
Adjunct Professor of Medicine
University of California,
San Francisco

An Overview Is a Meta-Analysis

During the past 15 years, "overviews" (as the British prefer to call them) or meta-analyses have been widely accepted as a powerful method for detecting small but clinically worthwhile treatment benefits. Most investigators consider a 10% survival advantage 10 years after treatment of cancer to be clinically worthwhile, especially if the toxicities of the treatment were modest. A benefit of that size, however, can be reliably detected only by a very large randomized trial. Although this is the preferred way to evaluate the effects of therapy, more frequently, multiple smaller trials are conducted because these are more easily administered and less costly to run. Most such trials, unfortunately, do not demonstrate a statistically significant benefit, even if there is a consistent trend.

Overviews can be used to circumvent the inadequate statistical power of small clinical trials by pooling the results of many smaller trials. In addition to detecting small but clinically worthwhile benefits, overviews provide greater statistical power, permitting evaluation of therapeutic effects in specific patient subsets.

Overviews of adjuvant tamoxifen (and adjuvant chemotherapy) trials were performed in 1985, 1990, and 1995. These clearly established that adjuvant tamoxifen could decrease breast cancer recurrence and mortality. Indirect comparisons of subsets within the overviews suggested that (1) longer durations of therapy were more effective than shorter treatment periods; (2) the effects of adjuvant tamoxifen were proportionally the same in all nodal subsets; and (3) patients whose tumors were ER-positive derived greater benefit than those with few or no measurable estrogen receptors. The results of the 1985 and 1990 overviews have been published,[1-3] but the 1995 report is not likely to be available until late 1996 or 1997.

In the Beginning: 1984

The first overview of adjuvant systemic therapy for early breast cancer was performed by Richard Peto, Rory Collins, Richard Gray, and the team from the Clinical Trials Unit of Oxford University in 1984. At that time, three randomized trials had demonstrated that the use of adjuvant chemotherapy might prolong the lives of premenopausal women with breast cancer.[4-7] No survival advantage had been observed, however, for postmenopausal women. Based on those data, a US consensus conference concluded that adjuvant chemotherapy should be standard for premenopausal women but not postmenopausal women.[8]

Europeans were more reluctant to use adjuvant therapy in any group of women because of its toxicity and because it seemed plausible that the effects of such treatment in premenopausal women might be entirely due to chemically induced ovarian ablation. Instead, European investigators designed a series of adjuvant endocrine therapy trials, the first of which was conducted in Denmark.[9] Americans, however, were skeptical about the likelihood that a cytostatic drug, such as tamoxifen, could destroy an adequate number of tumor cells to substantially and significantly prolong survival.[10] The first report, albeit only a brief letter to the editor of *The Lancet*,[11] that tamoxifen prolonged survival in patients with early breast cancer was published in 1983. Most breast cancer conferences on either side of the Atlantic during those years concluded with a debate between an American and a northern European, each espousing his or her particular perspective on this controversial subject.

By October of 1984, Richard Peto had successfully obtained the cooperation of every principal investigator of an adjuvant therapy trial, as well as at least some data from almost every known randomized trial conducted anywhere in the world up to that time, and had organized a conference to review results. Although investigators had submitted their data to the Oxford unit for analysis, none of those attending the conference had yet seen the results of the overview when they gathered at Heathrow Airport.

On the first evening, Peto outlined the goals of the conference and carefully explained the methodology, which was largely unknown to most of the investigators. It was clear that the techniques used for the overview analyses were potentially quite powerful. The next morning each trial was briefly presented. The tension and excitement mounted throughout the day until the results of the meta-analysis were presented in the afternoon. At the end of the presentation, there was no doubt in the minds of any but the most recalcitrant chemotherapy advocates that tamoxifen could not only prolong the recurrence-free survival of postmenopausal women with early breast cancer but could prolong overall survival as well. That evening at dinner, investigators placed small wagers on what the chemotherapy results would show on the next day. Many of the Americans suspected that the overview was a British trump card that they would use to win the ongoing debate once and for all.

Overviews can be used to circumvent the inadequate statistical power of small clinical trials by pooling the results of many smaller trials

The conference format was the same on the second day. Each of the chemotherapy trials was presented and discussed. At the end of the day, the overview demonstrated that chemotherapy also improved both disease-free survival and overall survival in postmenopausal women . . . to about the same extent as tamoxifen. During the course of the next year, these results were carefully checked and corrections were made. The analysis was again presented in Bethesda in September 1985 at another National Cancer Institute Consensus Conference. After hearing and reviewing the data, the consensus panel concluded that adjuvant tamoxifen should be considered standard treatment for postmenopausal women with positive axillary lymph nodes and ER-positive tumors.[12] Thus, the 1985 Overview put an end to the debate about whether adjuvant therapy prolonged survival. The principle had been established. A new era had begun in which research could now focus on how to improve the efficacy of adjuvant treatment.

By the time the data were ready for publication, however, it was clear that the first overview had overestimated the benefits to be derived from the use of adjuvant chemotherapy for postmenopausal women. The preparation of an overview is a tedious, detail-oriented project. Data must be checked and rechecked. The first analyses are not always consistent with the final publication.

How Is an Overview Performed?

The term "meta-analysis" has been used to describe a multitude of approaches to pooling data.[1] Many ignore the fundamental principle of an overview, which is to compare "like with like." Quality overviews are based on randomized, case-control, and cohort studies. The size and direction (positive or negative) of the effects of treatment are determined independently for each of the trials included in an overview, and these effects or benefits are then summated. Patients on the treatment arm are compared only with the patients in the control arm of the same study, never with patients in the control arm of another study. Beyond this fundamental principle, however, there are many legitimate differences of opinion about how to best proceed.

Some overviews include only published data or give greater weight to published data because they have undergone rigorous peer review and likely represent the highest quality studies. On the other hand, studies with a negative or null result are less likely to be published, and the exclusion of unpublished data introduces a different kind of bias. Some investigators perform their own quality analysis of studies and give added weight to those trials that meet certain pre-defined standards. The breast cancer Overviews utilize all available data, whether published or unpublished, and no adjustments were made on the basis of any factor, including perceived quality of the trial. As a consequence, the largest trials have substantially more weight in the final estimate of treatment effect than do smaller trials.

The first breast cancer Overview, performed in 1984-1985, included all randomized clinical trials of adjuvant systemic therapy that were initiated prior to January 1, 1985. Printouts of the data entered into the computers in Oxford were verified by each investigator. The validity of the randomization process in each trial was evaluated and any imbalances were investigated. In one instance, a trial was omitted because of questions about the validity of the results that emerged during a site-visit.

The first report on the 1985 Overview was published in 1988.[2] A very detailed report providing substantially more data and great detail on the overview methodology was subsequently published as a monograph in 1990.[1] A secondary review was conducted in 1990 and published in 1992.[3] No additional trials were added to this overview, but data from all the trials included in the 1985 Overview were updated through 1990. A third overview, which included all patients in trials initiated prior to January 1, 1990, was completed in 1995 and presented to the contributing trialists at a meeting in Oxford in September 1995. Although trialists are free to discuss this overview with colleagues and patients, no specific data from the overview are to be cited until all corrections are complete and the data are submitted for publication. Thus, only general observations and comments from the 1995 Overview will be included here.

1990 Overview

The 1990 tamoxifen Overview was based on 40 trials that enrolled 29,892 patients, 8,219 of whom had died at the time of the analysis. The preliminary presentation of the 1995 Overview included 58 tamoxifen trials that had enrolled 45,469 women, 15,257 of whom had died. Like a randomized trial, the real statistical power of an overview is derived from the number of events, such as recurrences or deaths, rather than from the number of patients enrolled. The number of events in these overviews far exceeds anything imaginable with one, or even two, large trials.

Expression of Results

The overview analyses are presented in one of two ways:[13]

As a reduction in the annual odds of recurrence or death. This is an expression of the proportional effect or the ratio of the effect of therapy in the treated compared to the control group.

As an absolute difference. This is the difference in the disease-free or overall survival curves on a life table plot at a single point in time. It is also referred to as the "rate difference."

The difference between the ratio and rate differences can be most readily understood by a simple example.[13] In Trial 1 presented in Table 1, 30 of the 100 patients randomized to the treated group and 40 of the

Table 1

Expression of Overview Results as "Ratio" Vs "Rate" Differences in Survival

| | No. of Deaths in Five Years | | Survival at Five Years | |
	Treated	Control	Treated	Control
Trial 1	30	40	70%	60%
Trial 2	6	8	94%	92%

| | Reduction In Mortality | |
	Ratio Difference	Rate Difference
Trial 1	25%	10%
Trial 2	25%	2%

In each of these two hypothetical trials, 100 patients were randomized to the control arm and 100 to the treated arm. Results at 5 years are presented. In the first of the two trials, 30 of the 100 patients randomized to the treated group and 40 of the 100 randomized to the control group died within the first 5 years of follow-up. Thus, at 5 years, 70% of the treated and 60% of the control patients were alive. This represents an absolute or rate difference of 10%. Another way to look at these data from the first trial focuses upon patients who died in the control group (N=40) or who might have died in the treated group. If treatment had no effect, it would be reasonable to expect 40 deaths in the treatment group. Only 30 deaths were actually observed. The 10 deaths that were prevented, divided by the 40 deaths expected gives a ratio difference of 25%.

Gelber RD and Goldhirsch A: The Concept of an Overview of Cancer Clinical Trials with Special Emphasis on Early Breast Cancer. *J Clin Oncol* 4: 1696-1703, 1986.

100 randomized to the control group died in the first 5 years of follow-up. Thus, at 5 years, 70% of the treated and 60% of the control patients were alive. This represents an absolute or rate difference of 10%. This represents the benefit from treatment for *all* treated patients, including patients who might not have died without the treatment. Another way to look at these data from trial #1 focuses entirely upon patients who died in the control group (N = 40) or who might have died in the treated group. If treatment had no effect, it would be reasonable to expect 40 deaths in the treatment group. Only 30 deaths were actually observed. The 10 deaths that were prevented, divided by the 40 deaths expected gives a ratio difference of 25%. This is not precisely the same as a calculation of the annual odds of death. Nevertheless, it is rough approximation and illustrates the difference between a proportional and an absolute survival benefit. (For a more complete explanation of this method, see reference 2).

Overall Results of 1990 Overview

All trials, worldwide, in which patients had been randomized to tamoxifen or no tamoxifen were included in the 1990 Overview. In some of these trials, women were randomized following mastectomy or lumpectomy plus radio-therapy to receive either tamoxifen alone or no adjuvant treatment of any type (Nil). There were other trials that compared tamoxifen plus some other therapy with the other therapy alone. Most often, these trials evaluated tamoxifen plus chemotherapy compared with chemotherapy alone. In general, the trial design was irrelevant. If there was a benefit from the comparison of tamoxifen versus Nil, there was usually a benefit from tamoxifen plus chemotherapy compared to chemotherapy alone. The size of the benefit might be different in the two types of trials, but the direction of the benefit (positive or negative) would be the same.

The overall result includes women from all age groups in trials that utilize a variety of different tamoxifen doses and durations of therapy. The reduction in the annual odds of recurrence or death and the absolute difference in recurrence or death at 10 years of adjuvant tamoxifen therapy are shown in Table 2. For comparative purposes, the results of the chemotherapy overview are also shown. No significant differences between the effects of adjuvant chemotherapy and adjuvant tamoxifen can be seen. (This is not necessarily true for all patient subsets, but that is beyond the scope of this discussion.)

Table 2

Comparative Reductions in Mortality (Proportional and Absolute), Chemotherapy Vs Tamoxifen

Therapy	Reduction ± S.D. In Odds Of	
	Recurrence	Death
Chemotherapy	21% ± 2	11% ± 2
Tamoxifen	25% ± 2	17% ± 2

Therapy	Absolute Difference ± S.D. At 10 Years For	
	Recurrence	Death
Chemotherapy	9.2% ± 1.2	6.3% ± 1.4
Tamoxifen	6.6% ± 0.9	6.2% ± 0.9

The effects of therapy described here are derived from overviews of all trials in which patients were randomized to either chemotherapy vs no chemotherapy (including trials in which patients were randomized to chemotherapy plus tamoxifen vs tamoxifen alone) or tamoxifen vs no tamoxifen (including trials in which patients were randomized to tamoxifen plus chemotherapy vs chemotherapy alone). All patients were included regardless of age or nodal status. The chemotherapy trials were limited to those that used at least several months of a drug combination; trials that employed a single agent and those that administered one course of chemotherapy (eg, perioperative trials) were not included. All tamoxifen studies, however, were included in the overview regardless of the duration of tamoxifen therapy or the receptor status of the patient. All differences are statistically significant with a p *at least* < 0.0001. Proportional = reduction in annual odds of death; absolute = difference in survival between the two groups at 10 years.

Early Breast Cancer Trialists' Collaborative Group, 1992: Systemic treatment of early breast cancer by hormonal, cytotoxic, or immune therapy: 133 randomized trials involving 31,000 recurrences and 24,000 deaths among 75,000 women. *Lancet* 339:1-15, 71-85, 1992.

ADJUVANT TAMOXIFEN: ANALYSES OF PATIENT SUBSETS

Age and Menopause

In the 1990 Overview, adjuvant tamoxifen was found to be less beneficial in younger women and premenopausal women (Table 3). Age appears to be at least as important as the patient's menstrual status, since the effects of adjuvant tamoxifen are nearly the same in women ages 50 to 59, regardless of whether they are pre- or postmenopausal. The effect of adjuvant chemotherapy in women younger than 50 is less than half as great as that of adjuvant tamoxifen, and again it makes no difference whether these younger women are pre- or postmenopausal. Nevertheless, these results must be interpreted

Table 3

Effect of Adjuvant Tamoxifen on Annual Odds of Recurrence and Death, by Age and Menopause Status

Premenopausal	No. of Patients	Reduction ± S.D. in Annual Odds of Recurrence	Death
AGE < 50	7905	12% ± 4	6% ± 5
50-59	1583	33% ± 7	23% ± 9
Postmenopausal			
AGE < 50	681	12% ± 15	(ZERO TREND)
50-59	7804	28% ± 3	19% ± 4
60-69	9452	29% ± 3	17% ± 4
70+	2656	28% ± 5	21% ± 6

This overview includes trials of tamoxifen vs no tamoxifen, including trials comparing tamoxifen vs no adjuvant therapy of any type, as well as those comparing tamoxifen plus chemotherapy alone in all age groups. Trials among older women were more often of the tamoxifen vs no adjuvant type, while among younger women, the trials were predominantly tamoxifen plus chemotherapy vs chemotherapy alone.

Early Breast Cancer Trialists' Collaborative Group, 1992: Systemic treatment of early breast cancer by hormonal, cytotoxic, or immune therapy: 133 randomized trials involving 31,000 recurrences and 24,000 deaths among 75,000 women. *Lancet* 339:1-15, 71-85, 1992.

very cautiously. Most of the trials evaluating tamoxifen in women older than 50 years of age were designed as "tamoxifen versus Nil." For women younger than 50, the trials more often compared tamoxifen plus chemo versus the same chemo alone. It is possible, therefore, that the effects of tamoxifen in women under age 50 might be much greater than shown by these studies.

In fact, this is quite plausible. Adjuvant chemotherapy causes transient amenorrhea in almost all premenopausal patients and permanent amenorrhea in the vast majority. Thus, it could be argued that the predominant effect of chemotherapy in younger women is a chemical oophorectomy. If this is the case, the combination of tamoxifen plus chemotherapy may really be a combination of two hormone therapies: tamoxifen plus oophorectomy! A comparison of the benefits of tamoxifen plus chemotherapy vs chemotherapy alone in women under the age of 50 to the benefits of tamoxifen vs Nil in women over the age of 50 would be inappropriate. Although combination chemotherapy has been shown in many randomized trials to be superior to single-agent regimens, this is not true for endocrine combinations. In multiple randomized trials, it has been impossible to show an advantage for such combinations.[14] (See discussion of 1995 Overview later in this chapter.)

Tumor Estrogen-Receptor Status

In patients with metastatic breast cancer, there is an excellent correlation between estrogen- and progesterone-receptor status and response to tamoxifen. This correlation would be expected to hold true in the adjuvant setting as well. An overview of all patients in all age groups, analyzed according to ER status demonstrated that adjuvant tamoxifen conferred a significantly greater advantage on those patients with moderately elevated or high levels of ER (Table 4).

It was surprising to find that the 1990 Overview showed a significant reduction in the annual odds of recurrence (13% ± 4) even in those patients who had ER-poor tumors; the reduction in the annual odds of death (11%, ± 5) was marginally significant. In fact, in women aged 50 and older, the reduction in the annual odds of death was significant in both patients with receptor-poor and receptor-rich tumors (16% ± 5 and 36% ± 3, respectively). Furthermore, in

Table 4

Effect of Adjuvant Tamoxifen on Annual Odds of Recurrence or Death, by ER Level

Receptor Level	No. of Patients	Reduction ± S.D. in Annual Odds Of	
		Recurrence	Death
ER - Poor or absent	5366	13% ± 4	11% ± 5
ER - Moderately elevated	11,733	29% ± 3	19% ± 4
ER - Highest Level	3174	43% ± 5	29% ± 7
ER - Unknown	9554	22% ± 3	15% ± 3
Test for Trend		p < 0.00001	p = 0.006

This overview includes trials of tamoxifen vs no tamoxifen, including trials comparing tamoxifen vs no adjuvant therapy of any type, as well as those comparing tamoxifen plus chemotherapy alone for all ER levels. Levels were defined by each trial group submitting data.

Early Breast Cancer Trialists' Collaborative Group, 1992: Systemic treatment of early breast cancer by hormonal, cytotoxic, or immune therapy: 133 randomized trials involving 31,000 recurrences and 24,000 deaths among 75,000 women. *Lancet* 339:1-15, 71-85, 1992.

the 1990 Overview, the effect of adjuvant tamoxifen in older women with receptor-poor tumors was greater than the effect of adjuvant chemotherapy in these women. This led many physicians to use tamoxifen in all older women, regardless of receptor status. However, the results of the more recent overview, described later in this chapter, should be noted.

Axillary Lymph Node Status

The *mathematical* interactions used to describe the relationship between a therapy and specific patient subsets may be qualitative or quantitative. In general, a qualitative interaction is one in which one group of patients derives benefit while another derives none. (It is important not to conceptualize "qualitative" and "quantitative" in terms of the non-mathematical relationship between therapy and a group of patients defined by pre-treatment risk factors.)

We might have anticipated that the interaction between tamoxifen and estrogen receptor status would be a qualitative interaction. However, qualitative interactions are quite rare in medicine. A quantitative interaction is one in which there is an effect of therapy in all patient subsets but the size of the benefit varies from one group to another. This is the most common interaction seen in medicine and the one that is applicable in most breast cancer analyses.

The quantitative effect of an interaction in two groups of patients with a different underlying risk of recurrence can be illustrated by a comparison of the two simple trials shown in Table 1. Patients in the second of these trials were clearly at a lower risk of recurrence: only 6 of the 100 treated patients and 8 of the 100 control patients died in 5 years. This resulted in 94% and 92% survival rates at 5 years, an absolute rate difference of 2%. The ratio or proportional difference is determined by assuming that 8 of the treated patients would have died if therapy had no benefit. Only 6 patients died. The 2 deaths prevented by treatment divided by the 8 deaths expected results in a 25% proportional or ratio difference. The proportional reduction in mortality is identical in the two trials. The absolute difference is five times greater in Trial 1, as shown in Table 1.

The interaction between tamoxifen therapy and risk, defined by number of positive lymph nodes, is almost identical to that illustrated in the example (Table 5). All patients regardless of age, receptor status, or duration of therapy were included in this overview. The reduction in annual odds of recurrence and death is not significantly different for those who had no lymph node involvement; one to three positive lymph nodes; or > three positive lymph nodes. The p value from a test for trend exceeds 0.1. The absolute benefits from the use of adjuvant tamoxifen, however, were greater in node-

Table 5

Effect of Adjuvant Tamoxifen on Annual Odds of Recurrence or Death, by Nodal Status

N 0/– refers to patients in whom no nodes were found at the time of either node clearance or sampling. N 1-3 and N 4+ refers to the number of lymph nodes found to have histological evidence of metastases from breast cancer at the time of either node clearance or sampling.

Nodal Group	No. of Patients	Reduction ± S.D. in Annual Odds of	
		Recurrence	Death
N 0/–	12,813	27% ± 4	17% ± 5
N 1-3	6053	33% ± 4	21% ± 5
N 4+	3941	26% ± 4	16% ± 5
Test For Trend		p > 0.1	p > 0.1

Early Breast Cancer Trialists' Collaborative Group, 1992: Systemic treatment of early breast cancer by hormonal, cytotoxic, or immune therapy: 133 randomized trials involving 31,000 recurrences and 24,000 deaths among 75,000 women. *Lancet* 339:1-15, 71-85, 1992.

positive than in node-negative patients (Figure 1) . Thus, the proportional effect of tamoxifen is the same in all nodal subsets while the absolute benefit is greatest among those with the greatest risk.

In clinical practice, which patient is more likely to receive a prescription for adjuvant tamoxifen: a postmenopausal woman with an ER-positive tumor and no axillary lymph nodes? Or a similar patient with eight positive lymph nodes? Figure 1 may be utilized to determine which patient is likely to derive the greatest benefit from adjuvant tamoxifen.

Few, if any, studies are large enough to allow analysis such as that shown in Table 5. Only an overview provides sufficient numbers of events and statistical power to which the method can be applied. Even in the performance of an overview, statistical power is rapidly spent when subsets of subsets are evaluated, such as analyses based on menopausal status, receptor status, plus number of involved axillary lymph nodes, for example.

OPTIMAL USE OF TAMOXIFEN: INDIRECT COMPARISONS

Dose

The overview data cited thus far have been derived from trials that used a variety of doses and durations of treatment. This is justified because the

FIGURE I Survival Overall (A) and recurrence-free (B) survival curves from tamoxifen overviews performed among patients who were either node negative or node positive. All

interaction between these factors and the benefits from tamoxifen are likely to be quantitative rather than qualitative. In other words, while both 2 years and 5 years of adjuvant tamoxifen therapy are likely to be beneficial, 5 years may be more beneficial than 2 years. Because of the enhanced statistical power achieved by combining both sets of trials, we can be more certain that adjuvant tamoxifen has an impact on patient survival, but an overview that combines these trials may actually underestimate tamoxifen's maximal effect when it is used optimally. Of course, the best way to determine the optimal dose or duration of tamoxifen is to conduct a randomized trial comparing two doses or two durations of therapy. Such trials are currently underway and results will be published in 1996. These data were not available, however, in 1985 and 1990.

patients, regardless of age, receptor status, tamoxifen dose, or duration of tamoxifen therapy, were included in this overview. From: Early Breast Cancer Trialists' Collaborative Group.[3]

When direct results from a randomized trial are unavailable, indirect comparisons may be made. For example, all of the trials that utilized 20 mg of tamoxifen per day might be compared with those that used either 30 or 40 mg per day. When this comparison was made for purposes of the overview, there was no discernible difference in the effect of tamoxifen, based on dose. Indirect comparisons of this type, however, are *never* as valid as direct randomized comparisons and should interpreted with caution.

Ideally, indirect comparisons should be used only to generate hypotheses that can subsequently be evaluated in randomized clinical trials. Indirect comparisons evaluating the optimal duration of adjuvant tamoxifen, performed in 1985 and 1990, have clearly had considerable impact on the use of adjuvant tamoxifen in clinical practice. (Unfortunately, warnings about the uncertainty of indirect comparisons that were included in the published reports of the Overview seem to have been largely unheeded by the medical community.)

Duration of Treatment

The first adjuvant tamoxifen trial, which was conducted by a group of Danish investigators in Copenhagen, administered the drug for 1 year.[9] Many subsequent trials also evaluated 1 year of adjuvant tamoxifen therapy. In the overview, these were grouped together as trials of "< 2 years." The first British trial, conducted by the NATO group (Nolvadex Adjuvant Trial Organization), utilized 2 years of tamoxifen, which led to numerous similarly designed studies. These trials were grouped together in the "2 years" duration-of-therapy category.[11,15] A third group of trials, the first of which was the Scottish adjuvant therapy trial, utilized 5 years of therapy,[3] although one or two trials used only 3 years. These trials were grouped together and classified in an overview as "> 2 years." Practically, the overview on duration of adjuvant therapy is a comparison of trials that used 1 year, 2 years, and 5 years of adjuvant tamoxifen. At the time these overviews were conducted, no data were available from trials in which patients were treated with adjuvant tamoxifen for more than 5 years. When all patients were evaluated together without regard to patient age, there was an unequivocal trend towards greater benefit

---

Table 6

Duration of Adjuvant Tamoxifen Therapy

The effects of adjuvant tamoxifen administered for 2 years, fewer than 2 years (mostly 1 year), and more than 2 years (mostly 5 years) were indirectly compared. This overview includes data on patients in all age groups and tumors from all ER categories.

Trials of Duration	Reduction ± S.D. in Annual Odds of	
	Recurrence	Death
< 2 Years	16% ± 3	11% ± 4
2 Years	28% ± 2	19% ± 3
> 2 Years	39% ± 4	24% ± 6
Test For Trend	1p < 0.00001	1p < 0.01

Early Breast Cancer Trialists' Collaborative Group, 1992: Systemic treatment of early breast cancer by hormonal, cytotoxic, or immune therapy: 133 randomized trials involving 31,000 recurrences and 24,000 deaths among 75,000 women. *Lancet* 339:1-15, 71-85, 1992.

Table 7

Duration of Adjuvant Tamoxifen Therapy, by Age

Patients were categorized as older or younger than 50 years of age and indirectly compared with respect to the effect of the duration of adjuvant tamoxifen therapy. As in Table 6, this analysis evaluated treatment for fewer than 2 years, 2 years, and more than 2 years.

Age and Trial Duration	No. of Patients	Reduction ± S.D. in Annual Odds of Recurrence	Death
AGE 50+			
< 2 Years	5730	19% ± 4	13% ± 4
2 Years	10,443	33% ± 3	23% ± 3
> 2 Years	5039	38% ± 5	23% ± 6
AGE < 50			
< 2 Years	2475	5% ± 7	4% ± 8
2 Years	4789	10% ± 5	4% ± 6
> 2 Years	1254	43% ± 11	27% ± 17

Early Breast Cancer Trialists' Collaborative Group, 1992: Systemic treatment of early breast cancer by hormonal, cytotoxic, or immune therapy: 133 randomized trials involving 31,000 recurrences and 24,000 deaths among 75,000 women. *Lancet* 339:1-15, 71-85, 1992.

with greater duration of treatment (Table 6).

The optimal duration of treatment appears less certain when subsets defined by patient age are evaluated (Table 7). While significant reductions in the annual odds of recurrence and death were seen among older women with any duration of adjuvant tamoxifen, 2 years of treatment were better than 1 year. There was no evidence from these indirect comparisons that 5 years of treatment was associated with significantly better survival than 2 years.

In contrast, although no significant benefit from adjuvant tamoxifen was seen for younger women when 1 or 2 years of therapy were given, a significant reduction in the annual odds of recurrence (43% ± 11) and a nearly significant reduction in the annual odds of death (27% ± 17) were observed in the trials that utilized 5 years of tamoxifen. Once again, these comparisons in the value of tamoxifen for older vs younger women must be interpreted with caution, since the trials in older women were primarily of the type in which tamoxifen was compared with Nil, whereas those in younger women were predominantly of the type in which tamoxifen plus chemotherapy was compared with chemotherapy alone. Taken together, however, these data support an important hypothesis: The optimal duration of tamoxifen may be different for younger vs older women. Firm conclusions regarding the optimal duration of tamoxifen, therefore, should not be drawn until adequate data are available from randomized trials in each of these age groups, and ideally, from trials that compare tamoxifen with Nil.

Combining Tamoxifen with Chemotherapy

To achieve maximum statistical power, trials in which tamoxifen was compared to no adjuvant therapy and trials that compared tamoxifen plus chemotherapy with chemotherapy alone have been combined. Among women aged 50 and older, this combined analysis included 29,892 patients; reductions in the annual odds of recurrence and death were 29% ± 2 and 19% ± 2, respectively. The majority of these women, 13,145, were in trials of tamoxifen vs Nil, and the reduction in the annual odds of recurrence and death were not much different than when the analysis was confined only to those randomized to tamoxifen vs Nil. This was not true, however, for younger women. Only 8,612 women under the age of 50 were randomized in tamoxifen trials of any type, and the reductions in the annual odds of recurrence and death were 11% ± 4 and 8% ± 5, respectively. Of these women, only 2,266 participated in trials that compared tamoxifen with no adjuvant treatment; when this subset was evaluated, there was a greater benefit associated with adjuvant tamoxifen. However, even then, the reduction in the annual odds of death (17% ± 10) among women aged 50 and younger did not reach levels usually considered statistically significant.

The trials in which a combination of tamoxifen plus chemotherapy was compared with tamoxifen alone in women over the age of 50 demonstrated a highly significant reduction in the annual odds of recurrence (26% ± 5); the reduction in the annual odds of death (10% ± 7), however, did not reach levels that could be considered statistically significant (Table 8). Of course, there was a highly significant benefit from adding tamoxifen to chemotherapy. This is not surprising, since tamoxifen alone was superior to chemotherapy alone in this age group.

Only 386 women under age 50 had participated in randomized trials comparing tamoxifen plus chemotherapy with tamoxifen alone world-wide by 1985! This is too small a sample size to generate any meaningful results, and thus in Table 8 the data for these patients are shown in parentheses.

In more than 6,000 women under age 50 who participated in trials that evaluated the value of adding tamoxifen to chemotherapy, tamoxifen added nothing in terms of either recurrence rate or overall survival (Table 8). Taken together, the overview shows very little, if any, advantage for combining tamoxifen and chemotherapy in either age group, especially if the outcome of greatest interest is patient survival.

Table 8

Tamoxifen Vs Nil; Tamoxifen Plus Chemotherapy Vs Tamoxifen Or Chemotherapy by Age: Effect on Recurrence and Mortality

Direct comparisons of the overview comparing tamoxifen vs no adjuvant therapy of any type (Nil) and indirect comparison of the overviews of trials in which patients were randomized to a combination of tamoxifen plus chemotherapy vs tamoxifen alone or chemotherapy alone, analyzed by age. Too few data were collected on women younger than 50 in the tamoxifen vs chemotherapy trials. These results are included in parentheses. All patients were included regardless of estrogen receptor status, dose of tamoxifen, or duration of treatment.

Tamoxifen Vs Nil	No. of Patients	Reduction ± S.D. in Annual Odds of	
		Recurrence	Death
AGE < 50	2,266	27% ± 7	17% ± 10
AGE 50+	13,145	30% ± 2	19% ± 3

Tamoxifen Plus Chemotherapy Vs Tamoxifen or Chemotherapy

AGE < 50			
Tamoxifen Alone	383	(32% ± 16)	(−6% ± 23)
Chemotherapy Alone	6386	7% ± 4	3% ± 5
AGE 50+			
Tamoxifen Alone	3930	26% ± 5	10% ± 7
Chemotherapy Alone	8099	28% ± 3	20% ± 4

Early Breast Cancer Trialists' Collaborative Group, 1992: Systemic treatment of early breast cancer by hormonal, cytotoxic, or immune therapy: 133 randomized trials involving 31,000 recurrences and 24,000 deaths among 75,000 women. *Lancet* 339:1-15, 71-85, 1992.

ADDITIONAL BENEFITS OF ADJUVANT TAMOXIFEN

Non-Breast Cancer Mortality

Although always referred to as an "anti-estrogen," tamoxifen is really an attenuated estrogen. Tamoxifen has been shown, for example, to exert estrogenic effects on the uterus in some animal species, and it is well established that tamoxifen can reduce cholesterol levels in humans. Evaluating these effects in breast cancer patients, however, is difficult. For example, it is difficult to determine the effect of tamoxifen on cardiovascular mortality because the vast majority of patients, especially those who are node positive and make up the bulk of the early adjuvant studies, die of breast cancer before cardiovascular disease becomes an important risk in their lives. As more patients with a lower risk are treated with adjuvant tamoxifen, however, the issue of cardiovascular disease will become more important. Similarly, the effects of tamoxifen on the incidence of uterine cancer are difficult to detect. Even a 25-fold increase in uterine cancer mortality or incidence among patients using tamoxifen would still yield a small number in absolute terms. Meta-analysis may be potentially enlightening with regard to both the cardiovascular and uterine effects of tamoxifen, but the 1990 Overview confined itself to questions related to non-breast cancer mortality and cardiovascular mortality. Endometrial cancer was not specifically addressed.

Among the 29,892 patients included in the tamoxifen overviews, only 429 of those treated with tamoxifen and 450 of those randomized to the non-tamoxifen trial arms died of any cause other than breast cancer. The number dying of causes other than breast cancer in the chemotherapy trials was even smaller (Table 9), which probably reflects the tendency to place higher-risk patients on chemotherapy trials rather than tamoxifen trials. A statistically significant reduction in non-breast cancer mortality is seen in the tamoxifen trials but not in the chemotherapy trials (Table 9). The reduction in mortality from vascular deaths (myocardial infarction and stroke) was more impressive: 25% ± 13 ($P = 0.06$). These data provide compelling evidence that tamoxifen has an estrogenic effect on cardiovascular mortality. This type of

Table 9

Mortality from Causes Other Than Breast Cancer: Adjuvant Tamoxifen Vs Adjuvant Chemotherapy

Deaths from causes other than breast cancer (ie, myocardial infarction, stroke) among all patients who participated in adjuvant tamoxifen and chemotherapy trials were compared. All trials and patient subsets were included. Control group patients in the tamoxifen overview did not receive tamoxifen, whereas those in the chemotherapy trials did not receive chemotherapy but may have received tamoxifen. Total of 990 non-breast cancer related deaths reported in paper. p = 0.05. More deaths were reported for chemotherapy as well.

| | Treatment | |
	Tamoxifen	**Chemotherapy**
Number of deaths observed: T/C	429/450	154/137
% Reduction in NON-Breast Cancer Mortality	12% ± 6	–4% ± 12
p Value	0.05	NS

Early Breast Cancer Trialists' Collaborative Group, 1992: Systemic treatment of early breast cancer by hormonal, cytotoxic, or immune therapy: 133 randomized trials involving 31,000 recurrences and 24,000 deaths among 75,000 women. *Lancet* 339:1-15, 71-85, 1992.

NS = not significant, T = treatment group, C = control group.

significant finding could not be demonstrated with a similar level of certainty by any single study.

Reduction in Contralateral Breast Cancer Incidence

When all tamoxifen trials were analyzed together, only 121 new cases of breast cancer in the contralateral breast occurred in women receiving adjuvant tamoxifen compared with 184 contralateral breast cancers in those randomized to no tamoxifen. This represents a 39% reduction in the incidence of contralateral breast cancer (Table 10). In addition, by the time of the 1990 Overview, it was evident that longer durations of tamoxifen treatment were associated with even greater reductions in incidence. In contrast, a similar analysis of the chemotherapy trials revealed no reduction in the incidence of contralateral breast cancer. Unfortunately, the number of events was still too small at the time of the 1990 Overview to evaluate this outcome measure separately for subsets of younger and older women. Finally, it will never be possible to determine from the overview whether this reduced mortality *from the second breast cancer*. That would only be possible with a very large (> 20,000 person) randomized trial in which tamoxifen is used to prevent breast cancer in women at high risk.

Table 10

Incidence of Contralateral Breast Cancer: Adjuvant Tamoxifen Vs Adjuvant Chemotherapy

The incidence of new breast cancers in the contralateral breast was assessed and compared among all patients in all adjuvant tamoxifen and chemotherapy trials. Control group patients in the tamoxifen trials did not receive tamoxifen, whereas those in the chemotherapy trials did not receive chemotherapy but may have received tamoxifen.

	Treatment	
	Tamoxifen	**Chemotherapy**
Number of contralateral breast cancers observed: T/C	122/184	40/42
% Reduction in incidence	39% ± 9	18% ± 20
p Value	< 0.00001	NS
% Reduction in incidence with durations of:		
< 2 Years	26% ± 21	—
2 Years	37% ± 13	—
> 2 Years	54% ± 16	—

Early Breast Cancer Trialists' Collaborative Group, 1992: Systemic treatment of early breast cancer by hormonal, cytotoxic, or immune therapy: 133 randomized trials involving 31,000 recurrences and 24,000 deaths among 75,000 women. *Lancet* 339:1-15, 71-85, 1992.

NS = not significant, T = treatment group, C = control group.

1995 OVERVIEW: WHAT'S NEW?

The results of the 1995 Overview have been presented in Oxford to the trialists who submitted data, as well as at many meetings around the world. These results must be considered preliminary, however, until they have been published in a peer review journal. For that reason, data have not been specifically cited from the 1995 Overview. Nevertheless, it is unlikely that changes in the numbers from that overview will have a material effect on the conclusions.

The single most important observation of the new overview is that the survival benefits associated with adjuvant tamoxifen that were seen during the first 10 years persist through 15 years— there is no evidence, in other words, that these curves begin to converge during years 11 through 15.

In addition, it is increasingly difficult to identify any single group of patients that derives *absolutely* no benefit from adjuvant therapy of one kind or another. In most cases, a combination of chemotherapy and tamoxifen is superior to either therapy alone. However, this fact illustrates a serious problem with the application of data from overviews to clinical practice. In the past, the finding that a particular therapy or regimen significantly improved survival in a randomized trial was almost always sufficient justification for use in practice. In the past, however, randomized trials were relatively small and had substantially less statistical power than an overview. Thus, only relatively large treatment effects yielded statistically significant results. That is no longer true. With large simple trials and, to a much greater extent, with meta-analyses, the physician must carefully evaluate the *size* and *nature* of the effect relative to any associated toxicities. Treatments that prolong life by only a few months may not be worthwhile to some patients, despite only modest toxicity.[16]

Tamoxifen in Women Aged 50 and Over

In the most recent overview, the effects of adjuvant tamoxifen in postmenopausal women continue to be substantial and greater than those associated with chemotherapy. Tamoxifen effects are seen in postmenopausal patients with ER-positive tumors, but also in those with ER-negative disease. Adding chemotherapy to tamoxifen still appears to confer additional benefits in older women, again for those with receptor- positive as well as receptor-negative tumors. Is this true for women over the age of 70? Probably not–but the numbers are too small to say anything specific.

Tamoxifen in Women Younger Than Age 50

There are now sufficient numbers of women under the age of 50 who have been evaluated in trials comparing adjuvant tamoxifen with no adjuvant treatment at all (ie, Nil) to more accurately assess the effects of adjuvant tamoxifen in this group. Among younger women with receptor-positive tumors, the effect of adjuvant tamoxifen is equal or nearly equal to that achieved with adjuvant chemotherapy. In contrast to the benefits of tamoxifen in older women, however, there is no effect from adjuvant tamoxifen in younger women with receptor-negative tumors. And, as had been reported in the prior overviews, there is absolutely no benefit derived from adding chemotherapy to tamoxifen in this age group. In an analysis of the effects of different durations of tamoxifen, no benefit was seen with just 1 or 2 years of tamoxifen, but a statistically significant reduction in the odds in recurrence and death was seen when more than 2 years of treatment were given.

Effects of adjuvant tamoxifen in postmenopausal women continue to be substantial and greater than those associated with chemotherapy

Additional Benefits of Tamoxifen

Not only is there continuing evidence that the use of adjuvant tamoxifen reduces the incidence of contralateral breast cancer, but also longer durations of tamoxifen have been shown to have a greater impact on the incidence of contralateral breast cancer than do shorter courses.

A reduction in non-breast cancer mortality was not, however, noted in the most recent overview. This must be interpreted cautiously. Many trials that were not included in the 1985 and 1990 Overviews are included in the most recent one. These new trials have had shorter follow-up periods. It is plausible that the effects of tamoxifen on non-breast cancer mortality might not be evident or might be obscured in shorter trials, since these events are more likely to appear with longer follow-up.

The most recent overview included an extensive analysis of the effects of adjuvant tamoxifen on second cancers, and it demonstrated that there was a highly significant increase in the incidence of *and mortality* from endometrial cancer. The absolute increase in both of these, however, was substantially less than 1%, and there is no evidence that the increase in incidence and mortality from endometrial cancer is sufficient to outweigh the benefits of adjuvant tamoxifen in any patient subset. At least one group has reported that adjuvant tamoxifen might increase the risk of developing colorectal cancer, but this was not seen in the overview.

Conclusions

Overviews of the adjuvant tamoxifen trials have provided important insights regarding the benefits of this modality and its appropriate place in the cancer specialist's armamentarium. Prior to the overviews, many experts seriously doubted whether adjuvant tamoxifen could prolong the survival of any group of patients. Thanks to sophisticated overview techniques, however, it is now clear that adjuvant tamoxifen has a substantially greater impact on the survival of postmenopausal women and about the same impact on the survival of premenopausal women with receptor-positive tumors as that seen with chemotherapy. Findings such as these have a profound impact on the practice of oncology, as well as calling into question fundamental assumptions about the relative effects of chemotherapy vs endocrine therapy. These data suggest, for instance, that there may be very little difference in the cytostatic and/or cytocidal potential of these two modalities, indicating that the magnitude of their tumor cell kill is about the same.

The decision to initiate tamoxifen prevention trials in both the United States and Europe was predicated, in large measure, on evidence provided by the overviews that non-breast cancer mortality and the frequency of contralateral breast cancers might be reduced with adjuvant tamoxifen. The fact that the absolute increase in endometrial carcinoma is trivial should be reassuring to most patients and physicians. No other source of information regarding such risk would be considered quite as solid as the tamoxifen overview. At the same time, the failure of the overview to show an advantage for adding tamoxifen to chemotherapy in premenopausal women demonstrates how these types of analyses can be used to avoid relatively ineffective treatment.

References

1. Early Breast Cancer Trialists' Collaborative Group: A systemic overview of all available randomized trials in early breast cancer of adjuvant endocrine and cytotoxic therapy. *Treatment of Early Breast Cancer, Volume 1: Worldwide Evidence 1985-1990.* p 207. Oxford: Oxford University Press, 1990.

2. Early Breast Cancer Trialists' Collaborative Group: The effects of adjuvant tamoxifen and of cytotoxic therapy on mortality in early breast cancer: An overview of 61 randomized trials among 28,896 women. *N Engl J Med* 319:1681-92, 1988.

3. Early Breast Cancer Trialists' Collaborative Group: Systemic treatment of early breast cancer by hormonal, cytotoxic, or immune therapy: 133 randomised trials involving 31,000 recurrences and 24,000 deaths among 75,000 women. *Lancet* 339:1-15, 71-85, 1992.

4. Valagussa P, Bonadonna G, Veronesi U: Patterns of relapse and survival in operable breast carcinoma with positive and negative axillary nodes. *Tumori* 64:241-58, 1978.

5. Bonadonna G, Valagussa P, Rossi A, et al: Are surgical adjuvant trials altering the course of breast cancer? *Semin Oncol* 5:450-64, 1978.

6. Bonadonna G, Rossi A, Valagussa P, et al: The CMF program for operable breast cancer with positive axillary nodes: Updated analysis on the disease-free interval, site

of relapse, and drug tolerance. *Cancer* 39:2904-15, 1977.

7. Fisher B: Adjuvant chemotherapy in breast cancer. *Int J Radiat Oncol Biol Phys* 4:295-98, 1978.

8. National Institutes of Health Consensus-Development Statement: Adjuvant chemotherapy of breast cancer. *N Engl J Med* 303:831-32, 1980.

9. Palshof T, Mouridsen HT, Daehnfeldt JL: Adjuvant endocrine therapy of primary operable breast cancer: Report on the copenhagen breast cancer trials, in Mouridsen HT, Palshof T (eds): *Breast Cancer—Experimental and Clinical Aspects.* pp 183-87. Oxford, Pergamon, 1980.

10. Henderson IC, Canellos GP: Cancer of the breast: The past decade. *N Engl J Med* 302:17-30,78-90, 1980.

11. Baum M, Brinkley DM, Dossett JA, et al: Controlled trial of tamoxifen as adjuvant agent in management of early breast cancer. *Lancet* 1:257-60, 1983.

12. Consensus Development Conference Report: Adjuvant chemotherapy for breast cancer. *J Am Med Assoc* 254:3461-63, 1985.

13. Gelber RD, Goldhirsch A: The concept of an overview of cancer clinical trials with special emphasis on early breast cancer. *J Clin Oncol* 4:1696-1703, 1986.

14. Henderson IC: Endocrine therapy of metastatic breast cancer, in Harris JR, Hellman S, Henderson IC, et al (eds): *Breast Diseases, Second Edition.* pp 559-603. Philadelphia: J.B. Lippincott, 1991.

15. Baum M, Brinkley DM, Dossett JA, et al: Improved survival amongst patients treated with adjuvant tamoxifen after mastectomy for early breast cancer. *Lancet* 2:450, 1983.

16. Henderson IC: Adjuvant systemic therapy for early breast cancer. *Cancer* 47:401-409, 1994.

Chapter 6

Tamoxifen for Adjuvant Therapy and for the Treatment of Advanced Disease in Premenopausal Breast Cancer Patients

Peter M. Ravdin, MD, PhD
Associate Professor of Medicine/Oncology
University of Texas Health Science Center
San Antonio

The last decade has seen a resurgence of interest in the use of endocrine therapy for breast cancer. New endocrine agents have been developed for the treatment of advanced disease, and the role of endocrine therapy in the adjuvant setting has been supported by new clinical trial evidence. An example of this increased interest in the use of endocrine therapy can be seen in the evolution of recommendations that have emerged from the St. Gallen conferences over the last decade.[1-3] In 1988, a summary of recommendations for adjuvant therapy by the international adjuvant therapy meeting at St. Gallen (Table 1) did not identify any subgroup of premenopausal patients for whom adjuvant endocrine therapy would be definitively the standard of care. This situation had radically changed by 1995, when endocrine therapy was included as standard of care or worthy of clinical investigation for several subsets of premenopausal patients. This chapter will address current views about the use of tamoxifen in premenopausal breast cancer patients.

Impact of the Adjuvant Therapy Overview Analyses

A role for tamoxifen as endocrine adjuvant therapy for premenopausal patients was not supported by the Overview analysis of 1985[4] (Table 2). Overall, the risk of death among premenopausal patients receiving adjuvant tamoxifen did not appear to be reduced. This result was not accepted as definitive, however, since some data suggested that premenopausal patients who received adjuvant tamoxifen without receiving additional adjuvant chemotherapy did indeed derive benefit. Another recognized important limita-

Table I

**Changes in St. Gallen Consensus Panel Recommendations
for Adjuvant Therapy in Premenopausal Breast Cancer Patients**

| | | March 1988 | | March 1992 | | March 1995 | |
		ER+	ER–	ER+	ER–	ER+	ER–
Axillary Node Negative	Low Risk	**None vs T**	NA	**None vs T**	NA	None vs T	NA
	Good Risk	ND	ND	**T**	NA	**T** C Ooph, LHRH-A	NA
	High Risk	**C**	**C**	**C ± T**	**C**	**C ± T** Ooph LHRH-A	**C**
Axillary Node Positive	Any	**C**	**C**	**C ± T**	**C**	**C ± T** **Ooph** ± T LHRH-A	**C**

Bold entries are treatments accepted for routine use or baseline in clinical trials.

ER = estrogen receptor, T = tamoxifen, C = polychemotherapy, Ooph = oophorectomy or ovarian ablation, LHRH-A = gonadotropin-releasing hormone analogue, NA = not applicable, ND = not defined.

tion of this early overview was that most patients had received fewer than 2 years of adjuvant tamoxifen treatment.

The second overview analysis in 1990[5] was somewhat more supportive of a role for adjuvant tamoxifen (Table 3). Again, premenopausal patients in unselected trials did not experience a net benefit with adjuvant tamoxifen therapy. In trials that were not confounded by the addition of chemotherapy, however, a trend for benefit with adjuvant tamoxifen was again noted. Although this trend did not reach statistical significance for survival, it was statistically significant for reducing risk of recurrence. Again, most of these patients were treated for 2 years or less with adjuvant tamoxifen. The notion that this duration of treatment might have been suboptimal was suggested by an analysis (Table 4) indicating that the duration of adjuvant tamoxifen appears to be important.

Oophorectomy Trials

A second line of evidence that appeared in the 1990 Overview supporting the efficacy of prolonged endocrine therapy in premenopausal patients was

Table 2

**Proportional Risk Reductions for Overall Mortality
Caused by Adjuvant Tamoxifen – 1985**

Subgroup	Patient Age	Number of Patients	% Reduction (Standard Error)
All Trials	< 50	3,418	−1% (8)
	≥ 50	10,465	**20% (3)**
No Concurrent	< 50	NG	21% (14)
Chemotherapy	≥ 50	NG	**19% (4)**
With Concurrent	< 50	NG	−9% (9)
Chemotherapy	≥ 50	NG	**22% (6)**

Data from the 1985 Overview Analysis.

Bold entries are statistically significant.

NG = not given.

the unexpected degree of benefit associated with oophorectomy. Individually, these relatively small trials had not appeared to strongly support the efficacy of adjuvant oophorectomy. Such trials were small by their very nature and were designed to detect only very large effects. Nevertheless, when analyzed together in the meta-analysis, it became evident that the proportional risk reduction afforded by oophorectomy in women younger than 50 years old

Table 3

**Proportional Risk Reductions for Overall Mortality
Caused by Adjuvant Tamoxifen – 1990**

Subgroup	Patient Age	Number of Patients	% Reduction (Standard Error)
All Trials	< 50	8,612	6% (5)
	≥ 50	21,280	**20% (2)**
No Concurrent	< 50	2,226	17% (10)
Chemotherapy	≥ 50	13,145	**19% (3)**
With Concurrent	< 50	6,386	3% (5)
Chemotherapy	≥ 50	8,135	**20% (4)**

Data from the 1990 Overview Analysis.

Bold entries are statistically significant.

Table 4

Effect of Duration of Adjuvant Tamoxifen Treatment on the Proportional Risk Reductions for Overall Mortality

Subgroup	Patient Age	Number of Patients	% Reduction (Standard Error)
Tamoxifen ≤ 1 Year	< 50	2,478	4% (8)
	≥ 50	5,735	**13% (4)**
Tamoxifen 2 Years	< 50	4,794	4% (6)
	≥ 50	10,496	**23% (3)**
Tamoxifen > 2 Years	< 50	1,311	27% (17)
	≥ 50	5,087	**23% (6)**

Data from the 1990 Overview Analysis.

Bold entries are statistically significant.

was 30% for recurrence, and 28% for death. This benefit was comparable to the 36% and 24% risk reductions for recurrence and death, respectively, that could be achieved by polychemotherapy in this group.

This result was made all the more provocative by the fact that the oophorectomy trials were carried out in an era in which the estrogen-receptor status of patients was not routinely assessed. These trials could be expected to have included, therefore, substantial numbers of patients who probably could not benefit from therapy. Using ER status to select patients for these trials might have resulted in even higher proportional risk reductions.

Scottish investigators reported just such a result in a trial comparing adjuvant CMF to ovarian ablation.[6] Although the two arms in that Scottish trial had the same overall efficacy, subset analysis showed that for ER-positive patients, oophorectomy was the superior treatment, whereas for ER-negative patients, CMF polychemotherapy was superior.

The 1985 and 1990 Overview analyses of adjuvant trials thus show that endocrine therapy may have an important role in the adjuvant treatment of breast cancer in premenopausal women, leaving unanswered some important questions about the use of adjuvant tamoxifen.

Duration of Therapy

The first of these questions centers on the appropriate duration of adjuvant therapy. That the duration of tamoxifen treatment is important is supported by the excellent efficacy of oophorectomy, which by its very nature is a

Table 5

Proportional Risk Reductions for Overall Mortality Produced by Adjuvant Oophorectomy

Subgroup	Patient Age	Number of Patients	% Reduction (Standard Error)
All Trials	< 50	1,817	**25% (7)**
No Concurrent Chemotherapy	< 50	878	**28% (9)**
With Concurrent Chemotherapy	< 50	939	19% (11)

Data from the 1990 Overview Analysis.

Bold entries are statistically significant.

prolonged endocrine therapy. Nevertheless, the numbers of premenopausal women who had received more than 2 years of tamoxifen adjuvant endocrine therapy were too small to define with narrow confidence limits the proportional risk reduction afforded by such therapy. Unfortunately, some of the most important studies addressing this issue included mostly or only postmenopausal patients, leaving the question of optimal duration of tamoxifen use in premenopausal patients largely unanswered. The 2-vs-5 years of adjuvant tamoxifen trial conducted by the Swedish Breast Cancer Cooperative Group, for example, which showed a significantly improved efficacy of 5 years of tamoxifen over 2 years, did not include premenopausal patients.[7] Likewise, the NSABP trial comparing 5 vs 10 years of adjuvant tamoxifen included primarily postmenopausal patients, and has not been analyzed by menopausal status.[8]

Confounding Effects of Adjuvant Chemotherapy

Another important issue in the adjuvant use of tamoxifen is whether the effects of the drug are less evident in patients who also receive adjuvant chemotherapy. The overview analyses from tamoxifen and oophorectomy trials suggest that this may indeed be the case in premenopausal patients. Thus, combined chemoendocrine therapy would not seem to be a preferred approach for premenopausal patients. This simple conclusion, while perhaps true overall, may depend on the type of chemotherapy given, the duration of the tamoxifen, and selection of patients. Some of the ongoing clinical trials may clarify this issue further.

Therapies for Low-Risk Patients

The value and limitations of adjuvant tamoxifen are suggested by the current Intergroup adjuvant therapy trial for low risk ER-positive premenopausal women, which randomizes women to tamoxifen alone or tamoxifen plus oophorectomy. Given that this population has an excellent prognosis (most were cured by their surgery), the average potential benefit from any therapy, in terms of increased average life expectancy, might be expected to be modest. Thus, only a low-toxicity regimen, such as an endocrine therapy, would be justified. In situations where the patient has a high risk of recurrence and death, however, current proportional risk reductions of < 50% are clearly very unsatisfactory, and more aggressive, even toxic, approaches are justified. This is why most ongoing clinical trials for patients at high risk for recurrence are focused on new treatment modalities, and new chemotherapeutic regimens, and not on what are expected to be only modest improvements with endocrine therapy.

Tamoxifen in the Treatment of Metastatic Disease in Premenopausal Women

One of the early concerns about the use of tamoxifen was that it might act on the hypothalamus and pituitary to block the negative feedback regulation of estrogens, which could result in supra-physiologic levels of estradiol. These high levels of estradiol might in turn overcome the anti-estrogenic effects of tamoxifen. Indeed, supra-physiologic levels of estradiol have been noted in normal women taking tamoxifen,[9] and in breast cancer patients during and after adjuvant therapy.[10] Total estrogen levels can rise to two to five times those that normally occur in nonpregnant premenopausal women. Because tamoxifen is thought to exert much, if not all, of its anti-neoplastic effect by reversible binding to the estrogen receptor, there is obvious reason for concern about whether high levels of estradiol might interfere with its action.

There is conflicting evidence about whether tamoxifen is less effective in premenopausal patients with metastatic breast cancer than in postmenopausal patients. In a large cooperative group trial examining predictors of response to tamoxifen in patients with ER-positive metastatic breast cancer (SWOG 8228), response rates were significantly lower in premenopausal women (24%) compared with postmenopausal women (57%).[11] Multivariate analysis in that trial showed that premenopausal status was an independent predictor of lower response rate, shortened time to treatment failure, and lower objective response rate. This trial, which included 342 patients, was the largest prospective study to address predictors of response to tamoxifen. Nevertheless, since only 37 of those patients were premenopausal, and the confidence interval for response rate to tamoxifen was quite broad, the authors felt that their conclusion—namely, that response rates to tamoxifen were lower in premenopausal patients—would need independent validation.

That tamoxifen and oophorectomy were associated with similar response rates (24% and 21%, respectively) in a trial randomizing 122 premenopausal patients to tamoxifen or surgical oophorectomy,[12] with no significant differences in time to treatment failure or overall survival, would seem to argue against the idea that tamoxifen is an inferior endocrine therapy in premenopausal women. A similar study of 53 patients who were randomized to tamoxifen or surgical oophorectomy also found no significant differences in response rate or survival between the two arms.[13]

Overall, tamoxifen is an effective agent for the treatment of patients with ER-positive metastatic breast cancer

If the elevated estradiol levels seen in premenopausal women treated with tamoxifen blocked or interfered with the drug's benefits, then one might expect an ovarian ablative regimen to be particularly effective in combination with tamoxifen. The concept of inducing total endocrine blockade by combining oophorectomy or an ovarian ablating treatment with tamoxifen is an interesting one. In general, however, studies have not shown major improvements in efficacy with such an approach.[14] Indeed, results of recent randomized trials suggest that no major benefit is to be gained by adding tamoxifen to an ovarian ablation over that which can be achieved with ovarian ablation alone.[15,16]

Overall, tamoxifen is an effective agent for the treatment of patients with ER-positive metastatic breast cancer. There is conflicting evidence as to whether tamoxifen is somewhat less effective in premenopausal women than in postmenopausal women, but if such a difference exists, it is relatively modest. Therefore, before cytotoxic therapy is initiated in an ER-positive premenopausal woman with metastatic disease, a trial of an endocrine therapy, such as tamoxifen, is nearly always indicated.

Safety of Tamoxifen in Premenopausal Women

In general, the side effects of tamoxifen are tolerated as well by premenopausal women as by postmenopausal women. Some of the best data in this regard (unconfounded by events due to cancer) come from the Royal Marsden Hospital pilot tamoxifen chemoprevention trial. These investigators reported that, relative to placebo, tamoxifen was associated with increased rates of hot flashes (36% vs 17%), vaginal discharge (13% vs 3%), and menstrual irregularities (22% vs 13%), but was not associated with increased rates of nausea, headache, or mood change in premenopausal women.[17]

Special considerations may be necessary when using tamoxifen in premenopausal women. For example, ultrasonographic studies have suggested than many premenopausal women develop ovarian cysts while on tamoxifen.[17,18] These cysts are generally asymptomatic, many are not clinically detected, and they often resolve after cessation of tamoxifen therapy.[19] Long-term use of tamoxifen by premenopausal women also seems to be associated with an increased incidence of uterine fibroids,[17] but, again, these rarely become clinically significant.

In contrast, some of the beneficial effects of tamoxifen may be less apparent in premenopausal women. For example, the presumably favorable effects of tamoxifen on serum lipids are more pronounced in postmenopausal women than in premenopausal women.[20] Also, although the use of tamoxifen seems to be associated with increased bone mineral density in postmenopausal women, paradoxically it is associated with a loss of bone mineral density in premenopausal women.[21]

Overall, however, tamoxifen is well tolerated by premenopausal women, with few patients developing toxicities that would require stopping therapy. Although the toxicities noted above may represent major issues for healthy women considering long-term tamoxifen as a preventive agent, they are less important for breast cancer patients contemplating 5 years of adjuvant tamoxifen, and of little consequence for women with metastatic breast cancer (given the much higher levels of toxicity associated with chemotherapy, and comparable or higher levels of toxicity associated with other endocrine therapies).

Summary

Tamoxifen is the best single agent for the treatment of breast cancer in premenopausal women who are likely to be responsive to endocrine therapy. It has a favorable toxicity profile, as well as high levels of activity in selected subsets of patients, both in the adjuvant setting and in the setting of metastatic disease. Its use may be optimized further by ongoing clinical and basic research designed to answer questions about which patients are likely to respond, what is the optimal duration of treatment, how to optimize use of tamoxifen in combination with chemotherapy in the adjuvant setting, and how to delay or prevent the onset of clinical drug resistance.

References

1. Glick JH: Meeting highlights: Adjuvant therapy for breast cancer. *J Natl Cancer Inst* 80:471-75, 1988.

2. Glick JH, Gelber RD, Goldhirsch A: Meeting highlights: Adjuvant therapy for primary breast cancer. *J Natl Cancer Inst* 84(19):1479-85, 1992.

3. Goldhirsch A, Wood WC, Senn HJ: Meeting highlights: International consensus panel on the treatment of primary breast cancer. *J Natl Cancer Inst* 87(19):1441-45, 1995.

4. Early Breast Cancer Trialists' Collaborative Group: Effects of adjuvant tamoxifen and of cytotoxic therapy in early breast cancer: An overview of 61 randomized trials among 28,896 women. *N Engl J Med* 319:1681-92, 1988.

5. Early Breast Cancer Trialists' Collaborative Group: Systemic treatment of early breast cancer by hormonal, cytotoxic, or immune therapy. *Lancet* 339:1-15, 71-85, 1992.

6. Anonymous: Adjuvant ovarian ablation versus CMF chemotherapy in premeno-pausal women with pathological stage II breast carcinoma: The Scottish trial. *Lancet* 341(8856):1293-98, 1993.

7. Swedish Breast Cancer Cooperative Group: Randomized trial of 2 versus 5 years of adjuvant tamoxifen in postmenopausal early-stage breast cancer. *Proc Am Soc Clin Oncol* 15:(abstract)171, 1996.

8. Fisher B, Digman J, Wieand S, et al: Duration of tamoxifen (TAM) therapy for primary breast cancer: 5 versus 10 years (NSABP B-1 4). *Proc Am Soc Clin Oncol* 15:(abstract)118, 1996.

9. Groom GV, Grilliths K: Effect of the anti-oestrogen tamoxifen on plasma levels of luteinizing hormone, follicle-stimulating hormone, prolactin, oestradiol and proges-terone in normal premenopausal women. *J Endocrinol* 70(3):421-28, 1976.

10. Ravdin PM, Fritz NF, Tormey DC, et al: Endocrine status of premenopausal node-positive breast cancer patients following adjuvant chemotherapy and long-term tamoxifen. *Cancer Res* 48(4):1026-29, 1988.

11. Ravdin PM, Green S, Dorr TM, et al: Prognostic significance of progesterone receptor levels in estrogen receptor-positive patients with metastatic breast cancer treated with tamoxifen: Results of a prospective Southwest Oncology Group study. *J Clin Oncol* 10(8):1284-91, 1992.

12. Buchanan RB, Blamey RW, Durrant KR, et al: A randomized comparison of tamoxifen with surgical oophorectomy in premenopausal patients with advanced breast cancer. *J Clin Oncol* 4(9):1326-30, 1986.

13. Ingle JN, Krook JE, Green SJ, et al: Randomized trial of bilateral oophorectomy versus tamoxifen in premenopausal women with metastatic breast cancer. *J Clin Oncol* 4(2):178-85, 1986.

14. Buzzoni R, Biganzoli L, Bajena E, et al: Combination goserelin and tamoxifen therapy in premenopausal advanced breast cancer: a multicentre study by the ITMO group. Italian Trials in Medical Oncology. *Br J Cancer* 71(5):1111-14, 1995.

15. Jonat W, Kaufmann M, Blamey RW, et al: A randomised study to compare the effect of the luteinising hormone releasing hormone (LHRH) analogue goserelin with or without tamoxifen in pre- and perimenopausal patients with advanced breast cancer. *Eur J Cancer* 31A(2):137-42, 1995.

16. Boccardo F, Rubagotti A, Perrotta A, et al: Ovarian ablation versus goserelin with or without tamoxifen in pre- and perimenopausal patients with advanced breast cancer: results of a multicentric Italian study. *Ann Oncol* 5(4):337-42, 1994.

17. Powles TJ, Jones AL, Ashley SE, et al: The Royal Marsden Hospital pilot

tamoxifen chemoprevention trial. Breast Cancer Res Treat 31(1):73-82, 1994.

18. Cohen L, Rosen DJ, Altaras M, et al: Tamoxifen treatment in premenopausal breast cancer patients may be associated with ovarian overstimulation, cystic formations and fibroid overgrowth [letter]. *Br J Cancer* 69(3):620-21, 1994.

19. Shushan A, Peretz T, Uziely B, et al: Ovarian cysts in premenopausal and postmenopausal tamoxifen-treated women with breast cancer. *Am J Obstet Gynecol* 174(1):141-44, 1996.

20. Ilanchezhian S, Thangaraju M, Sachdanandam P: Plasma lipids and lipoprotein alterations in tamoxifen-treated breast cancer women in relation to the menopausal status. *Cancer Biochem Biophys* 15(2):83-90, 1995.

21. Powles TJ, Hickish T, Kanis JA, et al: Effect of tamoxifen on bone mineral density measured by dual-energy x-ray absorptiometry in healthy premenopausal and postmenopausal women. *J Clin Oncol* 14(1):78-84, 1996.

Chapter 7

Additional Benefits of Tamoxifen for Postmenopausal Patients

Malcolm M. Bilimoria, MD
Research Fellow
Breast Cancer Research Program
Robert H. Lurie Cancer Center

V. Craig Jordan, PhD, DSc
Director, Breast Cancer Research Program
Robert H. Lurie Cancer Center

Monica Morrow, MD
Director, Lynn Sage Comprehensive Breast Program
Northwestern University Medical School

The benefits of tamoxifen therapy for patients with breast cancer have been established and confirmed. Results from the overview analysis show that postmenopausal women receive greater benefit from tamoxifen therapy with respect to disease-free and overall survival than premenopausal women.[1] In addition, tamoxifen causes a reduction in contralateral breast cancers, a finding that has led to prevention trials both in the United States and abroad. Tamoxifen has also been shown to maintain bone density and decrease morbidity and mortality from cardiac disease. These effects are a further rationale for the use of the drug in postmenopausal breast cancer patients who are not routinely given hormone replacement therapy (HRT).

A definition of the magnitude of benefit is essential in guiding physicians toward the proper duration of tamoxifen therapy. Previously, we have noted that results from several large clinical trials are needed to determine whether five years of therapy or longer is the best therapeutic regimen.[2] We concluded that the proven length of therapy would depend largely on the amount and degree of tamoxifen resistance within the heterogeneous clinical sample. Currently, tamoxifen trials in the United Kingdom are addressing whether 5 years of therapy or longer is the ideal regimen. In the meantime, each

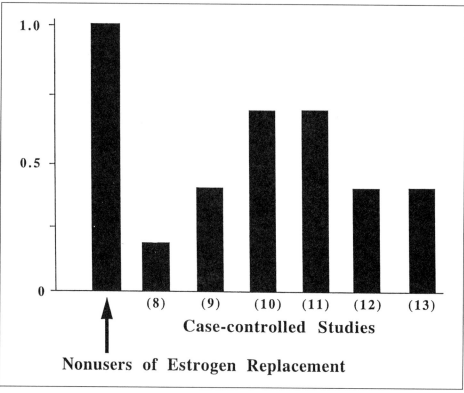

FIGURE I **Relative risk of hip fracture**   Relative risk of osteoporotic hip fractures in postmenopausal women who are nonusers of estrogen replacement (relative risk 1.0) compared with the relative risk in women on estrogen replacement therapy in six case-controlled studies.[8-13]

physician must weigh the benefits and risks of extending therapy beyond 5 years for each individual patient. This chapter will highlight the degree of benefit in preserving bone density and reducing cardiac disease that can be expected from tamoxifen therapy. In addition, we will analyze the extent of the reduction in contralateral breast cancers.

Menopause and Its Effects on Osteoporosis and Coronary Heart Disease

The majority of patients with early stage breast cancer can expect to be cured of their disease. Approximately 30% of patients with T1 and T2 node negative disease will die as a result of their cancer and only 10% of patients with tumors 1 cm or less in size will develop metastatic disease. Many of these women will be at risk of death from diseases associated with menopause, since a diagnosis of breast cancer usually prevents a woman from receiving hormone replacement therapy (HRT). Rosen et al[3] demonstrated that patients with node negative tumors less than 1 cm had a greater risk of dying from cardiac disease than breast cancer between 10 and 20 years post-diagnosis.

Osteoporosis is a major source of morbidity and mortality for postmenopausal women. Women begin to lose bone mass at about age 30; however, a significant acceleration of this loss (up to 5% per year) is noted after menopause.[4] It has been estimated that women can lose up to 35% of cortical bone mass and up to 50% of trabecular bone mass over their lifetime.[5] Population-based studies from the United States indicate that the lifetime risks of hip and vertebral fracture in postmenopausal, white females may be as high as 16% and 32%, respectively.[6]

Estrogen replacement has been shown to greatly reduce the degree of osteoporosis in postmenopausal women. An overview of hip fractures in current estrogen users showed that the relative risk is reduced to 0.2-0.7.[7-13] (Figure 1) Although osteoporosis is a long-term concern for postmenopausal women after a diagnosis of breast cancer, a more immediate problem is the risk of dying from coronary heart disease. It is estimated that, over her lifetime, a 50-year-old white female has a 46% chance of developing coronary artery disease and a 31% chance

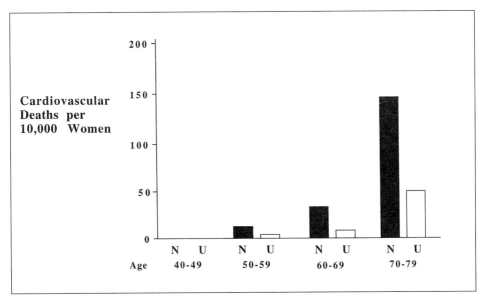

FIGURE 2 Cardiovascular deaths Comparison of cardiovascular deaths per 10,000 women in nonusers (N) and users (U) of estrogen replacement therapy for four different age groups. Adapted from Bush et al: *Circulation* 75:1102-1109, 1987.

Table 1

Effects of Tamoxifen on Bone Resorption

Study	Duration of Tamoxifen (Years)	Area Studied	Study Design	Control	Tamoxifen Treated Group	Statistical Significance
Gotfredsen	1	Distal radius	% change in BMC (g/cm)	−2.5%	−3.2%	NS
Fornander	2	Proximal radius	BMD (g/cm^2)	1.04	.99	NS
	2	Distal radius	BMD (g/cm^2)	.74	.70	NS
	5	Proximal radius	BMD (g/cm^2)	1.05	1.06	NS
	5	Dismal radius	BMD (g/cm^2)	.74	.78	NS
Fentiman	0.5	Femur	gHA/cm^2	.81	.81	NS
	0.5	Lumbar spine	gHA/cm^2	.95	.94	NS
Love	2	Lumbar spine	%/year change in BMD	−1.0%	.6%	p < .0001
	2	Radius	%/year change in BMD	1.29%	.88%	NS
Cuzick	6	Lumbar spine	BMD (g/cm^2)	.97	1.08	NS
	6	Trochanter	BMD (g/cm^2)	.75	.81	NS
Ward	1	Lumbar spine	%/year change in BMD	−2.3%	.09%	p = .04
	1	Trochanter	%/year change in BMD	−1.8%	1.4%	p = .03
Neal	5	Lumbar spine	BMD (g/cm^2)	1.028	1.059	NS
	5	Femur	BMD (g/cm^2)	.838	.894	NS
Turken	1	Lumbar spine	%/year change in BMD	−2.7%	2.4%	p < .003
Kristensen	2	Lumbar spine	% change in BMD	−4.3%*	2.5%*	p = .00074
	2	Distal radius	% change in BMD	−6.3%*	−2.0%*	p = .024

Adapted from Bilimoria et al: *Cancer J Sci Amer* 2:140-150, 1996, with permission.

NS = Not statistically significant, BMC = Bone mineral content, BMD = Bone mineral density, gHA = grams of hydroxyapatite.

*Percentages extrapolated from data graphs.

of dying from heart disease.[7] Sullivan et al[14] found estrogen use reduced the relative risk of angiography-detected coronary artery disease to 0.44, while Bush et al[15] found decreased rates of cardiovascular death for estrogen replacement users in nearly all age groups studied.(Figure 2)

Beneficial Effects of Tamoxifen on Bone

Initially, it was feared that the antiestrogenic effects of tamoxifen would actually accelerate bone resorption and increase the risk of developing osteoporosis. However, in vitro and in vivo studies have demonstrated quite the opposite effect. In one study, bone organ cultures pretreated with tamoxifen showed inhibition of bone absorption.[16] Ovariectomized rats treated with tamoxifen show a significant decrease in bone resorption compared to controls.[17]

The effects in patients on tamoxifen therapy have been equally impressive. Nine studies[2] examining the effects of tamoxifen on bone resorption are summarized in Table 1. Fornander et al[18] used a single photon absorptiometry technique to measure bone mineral density at the distal

Table 2

Effects of Tamoxifen on Lipoproteins

Study	Total Cholesterol (mg/dl)			LDL Cholesterol (mg/dl)			HDL Cholesterol (mg/dl)		
	control (# of patients)	TT (# of patients)	% change	control	TT	% change	control	TT	% change
Rossner	302(10)	258(11)	–15%	201	156	–22%	87	75	NS
Bruning	220(46)	205(46)	–7%	151	124	–18%	43	50	NS
Bertelli	254(36)	213(55)	–16%	180	127	–29%	55	56	NS
Bagdade	193(8)	204(8)	NS	122	115	–6%	45	49	NS
Love	216(70)	190(70)	–12%	138	110	–20%	57	53	NS
Ingram	259(47)	234(13)	–9%	193	171	–10%	66	61	NS
Cusick	256(47)	225(14)	–12%	186	145	–22%	50	43	–14%
Dnistria	244(13)	203(24)	–17%	169	123	–27%	55	56	NS
Thangaraju	224(45)	190(39)	–15%	149	132	–17%	54	58	7%
Saarto	237(26)	210(26)	–11%	154	122	–21%	63	60	NS
Average	249	214	**–13%**	165	134	**–19%**	57	52	NS

Adapted from Bilimoria et al. *Cancer J Sci Amer* 2:140-150, 1996, with permission.

TT = Tamoxifen treated group, NS = Not statistically significant.

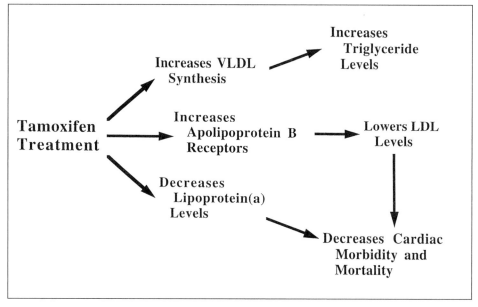

FIGURE 3   Lipoproteins   Effects of tamoxifen treatment on very low density lipoproteins (VLDL), apoliprotein B, and lipoprotein(a).

forearm in 75 postmenopausal breast cancer patients, and observed no increase in bone loss in patients taking tamoxifen for two to five years. Since then several studies have utilized the more sensitive dual photon absorptiometry technique to study tamoxifen's effects on bone density. Love et al[19] utilized this technique as part of a randomized placebo controlled trial of 140 postmenopausal breast cancer patients. Patients treated for two years with tamoxifen had a statistically significant increase in the bone mineral density of their lumbar spine when compared to patients receiving placebo. The five-year analysis of this same study supports the maintenance of bone density by tamoxifen therapy.[20] Seven other studies on both pre- and postmenopausal patients treated with tamoxifen confirm that bone mineral density is preserved or increased with respect to controls (Table 1). Three of these studies also noted preservation of trabecular bone at the femoral neck, a common site of postmenopausal osteoporotic fractures.

Beneficial Effects of Tamoxifen on Serum Lipids

When tamoxifen emerged as a proven therapy for breast cancer there were genuine concerns that treating women with an antiestrogen would adversely effect their lipid profile and lead to an increased risk of heart disease. Since then, several studies have shown that, much like tamoxifen's estrogenic effects on bone, tamoxifen also has estrogenic effects on serum lipid profiles. Analysis of nine separate studies reveals an average decrease in total cholesterol of 13% and an average decrease in LDL of 19% (Table 2).[2,21]

Love et al[22] in a randomized double-blind study of tamoxifen versus placebo noted increased synthesis of very low density lipoproteins (VLDL) leading to increased triglyceride levels and increased apolipoprotein B receptors, which resulted in lower LDL levels (Figure 3). Analysis at five years supports the maintenance of decreased LDL and total cholesterol.[23] Others have noted that tamoxifen interferes with cholesterol synthesis by inhibiting the conversion

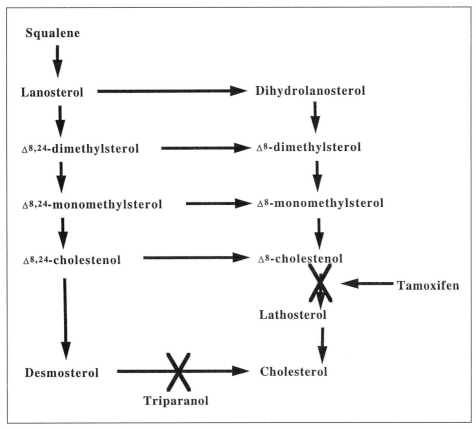

FIGURE 4   Schematic of squalene conversion to cholesterol   Tamoxifen blocks the conversion of Δ8-cholestenol to lathosterol, thus decreasing cholestrol production. It is important to note that tamoxifen does not cause a significant increase in circulating desmosterol. In the 1960s, a drug called triparanol was withdrawn from the market because it caused cataracts in patients after a few months of therapy. The drug blocked the conversion of desmosterol to cholesterol.

Table 3

Incidence of Contralateral Breast Tumors

			Tamoxifen Treated Patients		Controls	
Clinical Trial	Menopausal Status	Median Follow-Up, (Months)	Number of Patients	Number of Cancers	Number of Patients	Number of Cancers
NATO	pre & post	66	564	15	567	17
BCTC	pre & post	47	661	9	651	12
Rutqvist	post	53	931	18	915	32
Palshof	pre & post	78	164	3	153	4
Pritchard	post	70	198	3	202	3
Cummings	post	55	91	1	90	3
Fisher	pre & post	59	1419	23	1428	32
CRC	pre & post	40	947	7	965	18
Andersson	post	96	864	10	846	8
Ryden	post	108	239	11	236	15
Mason	NG	NG	367	4	1980	57
Total			6445	104	8033	201
				1.6%		2.5%

Adapted from Bilimoria et al: *Cancer J Sci Amer* 2:140-150, 1996, with permission.
NATO = Nolvadex Adjuvant Trial Organization, BCTC = Breast Cancer Trials Committee, CRC = Cancer Research Campaign, NG = not given.

of Δ8-cholestenol to lanosterol (Figure 4).[24] These metabolic changes are consistent with an estrogenic effect on lipid metabolism. Interestingly enough, high density lipoprotein (HDL) levels, which are usually increased by estrogen therapy, appear to be unaffected by tamoxifen therapy.

Beneficial Effects of Tamoxifen on Coronary Heart Disease

Tamoxifen's ability to lower serum lipids translates to a significant reduction in clinical cardiac disease. In 1991 McDonald and Stewart,[25] in a retrospective review of a randomized trial of tamoxifen versus placebo, noted that 10 of 200 women in the tamoxifen treated arm had died of myocardial infarction, while 25 of

251 had died of the same disease in the control group. An update of their patient data in 1995 showed that women in the tamoxifen-treated arm of the study had a rate of 14 myocardial infarctions per 1,000 years at risk compared to 23 myocardial infarctions per 1,000 years of risk for the control group.[26] Others have also found that longer durations of tamoxifen have a greater benefit in regard to cardiovascular disease. Rutqvist et al,[27] upon analysis of the Stockholm randomized trial, found that hospital admissions for cardiac disease were statistically lower for women taking five years of tamoxifen as opposed to women on only two years of the therapy.

Tamoxifen's ability to lower serum lipids translates to a significant reduction in clinical cardiac disease

The reduction in cardiovascular risk obtained from tamoxifen use appears to be mediated through the lowering of cholesterol levels mentioned earlier. It has been suggested that a 1% decrease in serum cholesterol results in a 2% decrease in the incidence of coronary heart disease.[28] Another possible mechanism for the cardioprotective effects of tamoxifen lies in the finding that tamoxifen-treated patients have a statistically significant reduction in serum lipoprotein(a) levels.[21] (Figure 3) Several epidemiologic and clinical studies have shown that increased lipoprotein(a) levels are an independent risk factor for coronary heart disease.[29,30]

Given that the majority of women with breast cancer are postmenopausal and that the number one cause of death in postmenopausal women (without a history of breast cancer) is cardiovascular disease, the lipid lowering properties of tamoxifen become clinically significant.

Beneficial Effects of Tamoxifen
in Regard to Contralateral Breast Cancer

Women with a previous diagnosis of breast cancer have a three-fold increased risk of developing a contralateral breast cancer when compared to age-matched women without breast cancer.[31] An analysis of 11 separate trials in a total of nearly 15,000 women reveals that the incidence of contralateral breast tumors in woman on tamoxifen therapy is reduced by 36% (Table 3).[2] In the 6,445 pre- and postmenopausal women who received adjuvant tamoxifen there were 104 (1.6%) contralateral breast cancers, while in the 8,033 patients randomly assigned to placebo or observation, contralateral breast cancers were present in 201 (2.5%). Though the trial patients vary with respect to stage of disease and menopausal status, as well as duration and dose of tamoxifen therapy, the chemosuppressive and chemopreventive effects of tamoxifen were evident in all of these studies.

Duration of Tamoxifen Therapy

Though tamoxifen has remained an integral part of breast cancer therapy for over 20 years, questions still remain concerning the optimal duration of therapy. As stated earlier, tamoxifen's benefits are not solely limited to its tumoristatic properties. These additional benefits must be taken into account when trying to determine the optimal duration of therapy for the individual patient.

The questions that need answering are two-fold. One, are the benefits of tamoxifen with respect to bone preservation and reduction in coronary heart disease maintained with longer duration therapy and will tamoxifen resistance or even tamoxifen-stimulated tumor growth effect morbidity and mortality in these patients?

As tamoxifen's estrogenic effects appear to account for the reduction in osteoporosis and cardiac disease and maintenance of bone density, much can be learned from the studies of estrogen therapy in postmenopausal women without a diagnosis of breast cancer. There is clinical evidence that the risk of hip fractures decreases with increasing duration of estrogen use. In one study, women who had taken estrogen for 1 to 2 years had a relative risk for hip fracture of 0.8 while women who had taken estrogen for greater than 10 years had a relative risk of 0.5.[32] Likewise, others have noted that longer durations of estrogen therapy result in decreased cardiac morbidity and mortality.[33] The non-cancer benefits of longer duration tamoxifen therapy become important in postmenopausal breast cancer patients who are long-term survivors of their disease. Many of these women, once they stop tamoxifen therapy, will be denied estrogen therapy because of their breast cancer history and therefore will be without any hormonal therapy to combat osteoporosis and heart disease.

With respect to tamoxifen resistant or tamoxifen-stimulated growth laboratory models exist demonstrating everything from complete tamoxifen stimulation to tumor growth that is noted only after tamoxifen is discontinued.[2] Clinically, the question of whether tamoxifen-resistant or tamoxifen-stimulated growth has an impact on survival is hard to answer because of the heterogeniety of tumors seen. Therefore, it is clear that an individualized approach to the duration of tamoxifen therapy is warranted. For example, a node-negative postmenopausal breast cancer patient with a family history of osteoporosis and cardiac disease may receive greater benefit from long-term (greater than 5 years) of tamoxifen therapy.

Trials designed to determine the efficacy of greater than 5 years of tamoxifen are currently underway in the United Kingdom. In the Adjuvant Tamoxifen-Longer Against Shorter (ATLAS) trial, women who have been on tamoxifen for at least two years and who, in conjunction with their physician, are

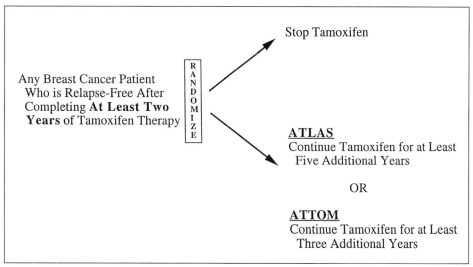

FIGURE 5   ATLAS/ATTOM   Study protocol of the Adjuvant Tamoxifen-Longer Against Shorter (ATLAS) Trial and the Adjuvant Tamoxifen Treatment Offer More? (ATTOM) Trial.

unsure of whether to continue are randomized to either stop tamoxifen or to continue for an additional five years. Most importantly, some patients are projected to be enrolled into a group of greater than 10 years of tamoxifen use.(Figure 5)

Additionally, the Adjuvant Tamoxifen-Treatment Offer More? (ATTOM) trial, is also underway in the United Kingdom. The trial is designed such that breast cancer patients with any nodal status and any ER status who have been on tamoxifen therapy for at least two years are randomized to either stop tamoxifen or continue for at least another three years.(Figure 5) Both the ATLAS and ATTOM trials will provide a huge database to answer the question about the appropriate duration of tamoxifen therapy.

Conclusion

At present, an insufficient data base exists to determine the proper duration of tamoxifen therapy, leaving the clinician and patient, after weighing the benefits and risks of tamoxifen therapy, to make this decision on their own for each breast cancer patient. In the postmenopausal breast cancer patient with early stage breast cancer, the benefits of tamoxifen therapy clearly extend beyond the tumoristatic properties of the drug. The bone cardioprotective effects of tamoxifen have been shown to decrease morbidity and mortality in these patients. In the end, the physician may have to individualize the decision by allowing those patients who stand to benefit the most from tamoxifen therapy to extend the duration beyond five years.

References

1. Early Breast Cancer Trialists' Collaborative Group: Systemic treatment of early breast cancer by hormonal, cytotoxic, or immune therapy. *Lancet* 339:1-15,71-85, 1992.

2. Bilimoria MM, Assikis VJ, Jordan VC: Should adjuvant tamoxifen therapy be stopped at 5 years? *Cancer J Sci Am* 2:140-150, 1996.

3. Rosen PP, Groshen S, Kinne DW: Factors influencing prognosis in node-negative breast carcinoma: Analysis of 767 T1N0M0/T2N0M0 patients with long-term follow-up. *J Clin Oncol* 11:2090-2100, 1993.

4. Cohn SH, Vaswani A, Zanzi I, et al: Effect of aging on bone mass in adult women. *Am J Physiol* 230:143-147, 1976.

5. Lobo RA, Pickar JH, Wild RA, et al: Metabolic impact of adding medroxyprogesterone acetate to conjugated estrogen therapy in postmenopausal women. *Obstet Gynecol* 84:987-995, 1994.

6. Cummings SR, Black DM, Rubin SM: Lifetime risks of hip, Collesi or vertebral fractures and coronary heart disease among white postmenopausal women. *Ann Int Med* 149:2445-2450, 1989.

7. Grady D, Rubin SM, Pettiti DB, et al: Hormone therapy to prevent disease and prolong life in postmenopausal women. *Ann Int Med* 117:1016-1037, 1992.

8. Hutchinson TA, Polansky SM, Feinstein AR: Post-menopausal oestrogens protect against fractures of hip and distal radius: A case-control study. *Lancet* 2:705-709, 1979.

9. Weiss NS, Ure CL, Ballard JH: Decreased risk of fractures of the hip and lower forearm with postmenopausal use of estrogen. *N Engl J Med* 303:1195-1198, 1980.

10. Johnson RE, Specht EE: The risk of hip fracture in postmenopausal females with and without estrogen drug exposure. *Am J Public Health* 71:138-144, 1981.

11. Paganini-Hill A, Ross RK, Gerkins VR, et al: Menopausal estrogen therapy and hip fractures. *Ann Intern Med* 95:28-31, 1981.

12. Kreiger N, Kelsey JL, Holford TR: An epidemiologic study of hip fracture in postmenopausal women. *Am J Epidemiol* 116:141-148, 1982.

13. Williams AR, Weiss NS, Ure CL: Effect of weight, smoking, and estrogen use on the risk of hip and forearm fractures in postmenopausal women. *Obstet Gynecol* 60:695-699, 1982.

14. Sullivan JM, VanderZwaag R, Lemp UF: Postmenopausal estrogen use and coronary atherosclerosis. *Ann Int Med* 108:358-363, 1988.

15. Bush TL, Barrett-Connor E, Cowan LD, et al: Cardiovascular mortality and noncontraceptive use of estrogen in women: Results from the Lipid Research Clinics Program Follow-up Study. *Circulation* 75:1102-1109, 1987.

16. Stewart PJ, Stern PH: Effects of antiestrogens, tamoxifen, and clomiphene on bone resorption in vitro. *Endocrinology* 118:125-131, 1986.

17. Jordan VC, Phelps E, Lindgren UJ: Effects of antiestrogens on bone in castrated and intact female rats. *Breast Cancer Res Treat* 10:31-35, 1987.

18. Fornander T, Rutqvist LE, Sjoberg HE, et al: Long-term adjuvant tamoxifen in early breast cancer: effect on bone mineral density in postmenopausal women. *J Clin Oncol* 8:1019-1024, 1990.

19. Love RR, Mazess RB, Barden HS, et al: Effects of tamoxifen on bone mineral density in postmenopausal women with breast cancer. *N Engl J Med* 326:852-856, 1992.

20. Love RR, Barden HS, Mazess RB: Effect of tamoxifen on lumbar spine bone mineral density in postmenopausal women after 5 years. *Arch Int Med* 154:2585-2588, 1994.

21. Saarto T, Blomqvist C, Ehnholm C: Antiatherogenic effects of adjuvant antiestrogens: A randomized trial comparing the effects of tamoxifen and toremifene on plasma lipid levels in postmenopausal women with node-positive breast cancer. *J Clin Oncol* 14:429-433, 1996.

22. Love RR, Wiebe D, Newcomb P, et al: Effects of tamoxifen on cardiovascular risk factors in postmenopausal women. *Ann Intern Med* 115:860-864, 1991.

23. Love RR, Wiebe DA, Feyzi JM: Effects of tamoxifen on cardiovascular risk factors in postmenopausal women after 5 years of treatment. *J Natl Cancer Inst* 86:1534-1539, 1994.

24. Gylling H, Pyrhonen S, Mantyla E: Tamoxifen and toremifene lower serum cholesterol by inhibition of $\Delta 8$-cholestenol conversion to lathosterol in women with breast cancer. *J Clin Oncol* 13:2900-2905, 1995.

25. McDonald CC, Stewart HJ: Fatal myocardial infarctions in the Scottish adjuvant tamoxifen trial. *Br Med J* 303:435-437, 1991.

26. McDonald CC, Alexander FE, Whyte BW, et al: Cardiac and vascular morbidity in women receiving adjuvant tamoxifen for breast cancer in a randomised trial. *Br Med J* 311:977-980, 1995.

27. Rutqvist LE, Mattsson A: Cardiac and thromboembolic morbidity among postmenopausal women with early stage breast cancer in a randomized trial of adjuvant tamoxifen. *J Natl Cancer Inst* 85:1398-1406, 1993.

28. Castelli WP: Cholesterol and lipids in the risk of coronary artery disease—the Framingham Heart Study. *Canad J Card* 4:5A-10A, 1988.

29. Loscalzo J: Lipoprotein(a): A unique risk factor for atherothrombotic disease. *Arteriosclerosis* 10:672-679, 1990.

30. Utermann G: Lipoprotein(a): A genetic risk factor for premature coronary heart disease. *Curr Opin Lipidol* 1:404-410, 1990.

31. Boring C, Squire T, Tong T, et al: Cancer Statistics. *CA Cancer J Clin* 44:7-26, 1994.

32. Weiss NS, Ure CL, Ballard JH: Decreased risks of fractures of the hip and lower forearm with postmenopausal use of estrogen. *N Engl J Med* 303:1044-1049, 1980.

33. Gorsky RD, Koplan JP, Peterson HB, et al: Relative risks and benefits of long-term estrogen replacement therapy: A decision analysis. *Obstet Gynecol* 83:161-166, 1994.

Chapter 8

Controversies on the Duration of Tamoxifen Administration in the Adjuvant Setting

Norman Wolmark, MD
Chairman, Department of Human Oncology
Medical College of Pennsylvania/Hahnemann University
Allegheny Campus, Pittsburgh
Chairman, National Surgical Breast and Bowel Project (NSABP)

Over the past 2 decades, there has been an accumulating database demonstrating that tamoxifen used in the adjuvant setting for stage I and II breast cancer results in an unequivocal prolongation in disease-free survival and overall survival. What is considerably less apparent is the optimal duration for the administration of tamoxifen. On November 30, 1995, the National Cancer Institute issued a clinical announcement,[1] based in large part on data from the National Surgical Adjuvant Breast and Bowel Project (NSABP) protocol B-14, in which it was concluded that there was no advantage for continuation of tamoxifen beyond 5 years in women with node-negative estrogen-receptor positive breast cancers. The casual observer with an interest in breast cancer, who is not directly involved in clinical trials, might appropriately ask why it has taken 20 years to address a question as basic as the duration of treatment for the most commonly used agent in the management of breast cancer. In an effort to respond to this hypothetical question, it might be of interest to review the sequence of NSABP protocols in the adjuvant setting, since invariably this sequence is reflective of the rationale and beliefs that were then extant outside the context of clinical trials. This exercise provides a historical perspective and a partial explanation for the rather convoluted approach that was evolved to determine the optimum duration of tamoxifen therapy.

The first NSABP randomized prospective clinical trial addressing the value of adjuvant therapy in breast cancer was initiated in 1972. The initial series of trials all assessed various chemotherapeutic regimens administered with the rationale that chemotherapy, given in the postoperative setting, would eradicate established micro-metastases and prolong survival. Because it was hypothesized that patients with histologically positive nodes were more likely to harbor micro-metastases at the time of operation, the first generation of NSABP trials was limited to women with histologically positive nodes.

When it became apparent that adjuvant chemotherapy was of benefit in this patient population, adjuvant chemotherapy was elevated to the status of standard therapy and consequently became the baseline against which the efficacy of tamoxifen would be measured. As a direct result of this event, when the NSABP initiated its first clinical trial assessing the utility of tamoxifen in the adjuvant setting in 1978, protocol B-09, it was carried out in an environment where all patients received chemotherapy, the standard of the day. The NSABP chemotherapeutic regimen at that time consisted of L-PAM and 5-FU given for a period of 2 years.[2] The duration of tamoxifen administration was empirically chosen to coincide with the period of chemotherapy administration. Patients with histologically positive nodes were randomized to receive either chemotherapy alone or chemotherapy together with 2 years of tamoxifen; a recent analysis of the results after 12 years of follow-up indicates that "tamoxifen responsive" patients, a group largely comprised of women > 49 years of age, had a highly significant prolongation in disease-free survival and survival as a result of the addition of tamoxifen. While NSABP protocol B-09 was accruing patients, it was already appreciated that the 2-year period selected for tamoxifen administration might not represent the optimal regimen.

Accordingly, following the closure of patient accession in 1980, an additional group of patients with similar "tamoxifen responsive" characteristics were all treated with L-PAM, 5-FU and tamoxifen, only in this latter patient population, the tamoxifen was given for a total period of 3 years. Thus, there was an opportunity, albeit an indirect one, to compare the effects of 2 years of tamoxifen to 3 years of tamoxifen when added to a chemotherapy baseline in patients with positive nodes.[3] The results from this study indicate that at 8 years of follow-up there was a disease-free survival and overall survival advantage for the group receiving 3 years of tamoxifen; this advantage has become attenuated, however, by the 10th year of follow-up and is no longer statistically significant.

By the early 1980s, after the first decade of clinical trials assessing adjuvant therapy in stage II breast cancer had elapsed, it was believed that women < 50 years of age sustained the greatest benefit from adjuvant chemotherapy and women > 49 years of age benefited from tamoxifen-containing regimens. Preliminary evidence also suggested that 3 years of tamoxifen added to chemotherapy was superior to 2 years and that, perhaps, longer duration of treatment would be translated into further incremental gains. It became increasingly apparent that in "tamoxifen responsive" women with histologically positive nodes, the role of tamoxifen, used alone without chemotherapy, had not yet been determined. It was argued at that time that the benefits attributable to L-PAM and 5-FU in women > 49 years of age were, at best, modest. It was further postulated that the advantages obtained by the combination of L-PAM, 5-FU and tamoxifen might have been achieved by the administration of tamoxifen alone without chemotherapy. Accordingly, the NSABP made the decision to retrace its steps: A study was introduced that compared the combination of chemotherapy plus tamoxifen to tamoxifen alone in women > 49 years age with histologically positive nodes. Protocol B-16 was initiated in October of 1984 and approximately 1,300 patients were randomized to receive one of three treatment options:[4]

The duration of tamoxifen administration was empirically chosen to coincide with the period of chemotherapy administration

- Tamoxifen alone
- Adriamycin, cyclophosphamide and tamoxifen or
- L-PAM, 5-FU (with or without Adriamycin) together with tamoxifen.

A pair-wise comparison between the group receiving tamoxifen alone and patients receiving the combination of Adriamycin/cyclophosphamide plus tamoxifen indicates that tamoxifen in combination with chemotherapy is significantly superior to tamoxifen alone relative to disease-free survival and overall survival at 7 years of follow-up. This study was one of the first to demonstrate an unequivocal benefit for chemotherapy when used in a population of women > 49 years of age; further, it demonstrated that the concomitant addition of tamoxifen to chemotherapy was superior to tamoxifen alone in this population.

As a result of these findings, Adriamycin/cyclophosphamide and tamoxifen became the NSABP standard for this patient cohort in subsequent trials. The duration of tamoxifen administration, at the beginning of this study in 1984, was established at 4 years, a determination based more upon empiricism than fact. The definitive test for assessing the optimal duration of tamoxifen administration would be conducted in a setting where tamoxifen could be used as a single agent in node-negative patients.

Because of the prevalent belief during the 1970s that the risk of chemotherapy prohibited its investigation in node-negative patients who allegedly had a good prognosis, it was not until 1981, despite several prior attempts, that the NSABP was able to initiate two clinical trials evaluating adjuvant therapy in patients with negative nodes: NSABP protocols B-13 and B-14. NSABP protocol B-13 was restricted to node-negative patients whose tumors

were receptor negative; 760 patients were randomized to receive no chemotherapy or sequential methotrexate and 5-FU.[5] This regimen was selected
because it was considered inappropriate to use an alkylating agent with a
putative leukemogenic potential in a good risk population, a conclusion that
subsequently could not be substantiated. Results through 7 years of follow-up
showed a significant disease-free survival benefit for women < 50 years of age
as well as those > 49 years. Concomitant with the start of protocol B-13,
protocol B-14 was commenced in women with histologically negative nodes
whose tumors were receptor positive (≥ 10 fmol); patients were randomized
to receive either tamoxifen or a placebo and a potential setting was finally
provided where a definitive assessment of duration of tamoxifen administration could be carried out.

At the start of this study in January of 1982, however, the question of
tamoxifen duration was not addressed and originally tamoxifen was to have
been administered for 2 years. As the proponents of prolonged tamoxifen
administration became more numerous and outspoken (unencumbered by
data), the trial was modified so that tamoxifen was to be given for a period of
5 years. It was not until 1986, that the decision was made to modify protocol B-
14 in order to compare 5 years of tamoxifen with 10 years of tamoxifen.
Because the NCI-generated clinical announcement on the duration of tamoxifen therapy[1] relied heavily on data from NSABP protocol B-14, it would
seem appropriate to review this trial in some detail.

NSABP Protocol B-14: Study Rationale and Conduct

This study was limited to patients with primary breast cancer and histologically negative axillary nodes whose tumor estrogen receptors were positive
(≥ 10 fmol). Following either mastectomy or lumpectomy, patients were
randomized to receive either 5 years of tamoxifen or 5 years of placebo;
patients who were initially treated with lumpectomy received postoperative
radiotherapy to the ipsilateral breast together with tamoxifen or placebo
administration. There are two basic components associated with this trial; the
first and principal component ("principal randomization") was formulated to
determine whether patients who received tamoxifen had a superior disease-
free survival and overall survival compared with those patients who were
randomized to receive a placebo (Figure 1). This part of the study was
initiated in January of 1982; randomization was closed in January of 1988 after
2,818 eligible patients had been entered. The "second randomization" was
initiated in 1987, after the decision had been made to modify the trial to
address the tamoxifen duration question. This latter part of the study, therefore, was designed to compare the efficacy of 5 years of tamoxifen treatment

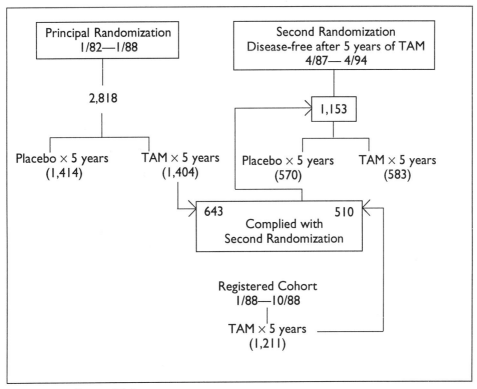

FIGURE 1 Protocol Schemas

with 10 years of tamoxifen treatment. Patients eligible for this "second randomization" were derived from two patient populations: those women who had initially been randomized into protocol B-14 who had completed the assigned 5 years of tamoxifen treatment, remained free of breast cancer recurrence, and who agreed to participate were rerandomized to either an additional 5 years of tamoxifen or 5 years of placebo in a double-blinded fashion. Patients who had been randomized to a placebo in the initial component of this trial were not eligible for the second randomization.

It became evident that to achieve sufficient power to answer the duration question, additional patients who had all received 5 years of tamoxifen would need to be recruited. For this reason, between January of 1988 and October of 1988, an additional 1,211 eligible patients who fulfilled the same criteria were registered to receive 5 years of tamoxifen ("registered cohort"). Patients in this cohort who were free of cancer recurrence at 5 years were offered the second randomization to an additional 5 years of tamoxifen or an additional 5 years of placebo. Thus, between 1987 and 1994, there were 1,153 eligible patients who were disease free after 5 years of tamoxifen and who agreed to be rerandomized; 55% of this population was derived from the original tamoxifen patient population and 45% entered the second randomization as part of the "registered cohort." Patient characteristics were similar among all subjects. In all components of the study, those patients who were randomized to receive tamoxifen were treated with 10 mg bid. Of these 1,153 patients, approximately 57% were treated with total mastectomy and 43% with a breast -preserving procedure followed by radiotherapy. The results from both components of protocol B-14 were published in the latter part of 1996[6].

Results: Tamoxifen vs Placebo—Principal Randomization

It is important not to confuse the results from the "second randomization" comparing 5 vs 10 years of tamoxifen with those from the first component of the trial addressing the principal aim, namely, whether tamoxifen is superior to placebo in node-negative receptor-positive patients (principal randomization). Four-year results comparing tamoxifen to placebo were first reported in 1989,[7] at which time there was a significant disease-free survival and a borderline survival advantage in favor of tamoxifen-treated patients; the results now at 10 years confirm and extend the conclusions of the initial analyses performed at 4 years (Table 1). The tamoxifen group includes those patients who stopped treatment after 5 years as well as those who continued tamoxifen as part of the second randomization. There is a highly significant prolongation in disease-free survival, 69% vs 57%, in favor of the tamoxifen-treated group ($P < 0.0001$). This difference in disease-free survival is reflected in a similar advantage in distant disease-free survival, 76% vs 67%, ($P < 0.0001$) and overall survival, 80% vs 76% ($P = 0.02$). This analysis is limited to the patients randomized to tamoxifen or placebo between 1982 and 1988 (see Table 1).

Table I

**Principal Randomization:
Tamoxifen vs Placebo**

	Tamoxifen	Placebo	P
DFS	69%	57%	< 0.0001
DDFS	76%	69%	< 0.0001
S	80%	76%	0.02

DFS = disease-free survival, DDFS = distant disease-free survival, S = survival.

At 10 years, the incidence of tumor recurrence within the ipsilateral breast was 10.3% for the placebo-treated patients compared with 3.4% for those treated with tamoxifen. That the benefits of tamoxifen therapy are not limited to local and regional disease is clearly demonstrated by the highly significant differences in distant disease-free survival and overall survival. The reduction in the occurrence of contralateral breast cancer attributable to tamoxifen in the original report of the data is still apparent at 10 years. The cumulative incidence of contralateral breast tumor occurrence at 10 years is 3.8% in tamoxifen-treated patients and 6.1% for patients randomized to the placebo arm (56 vs 82 events). The advantage associated with tamoxifen was not related to the age of the patient; patients who were < 50 years of age derived a benefit at least as great as those > 49 years.

Adverse Effects and Endometrial Cancer (Principal Randomization)

Hot flashes, vaginal discharge, and irregular menses were more frequent in women who were treated with tamoxifen, whereas fluid retention and weight gain were similar in the placebo and the tamoxifen-treated groups. Thromboembolic phenomena were higher in the tamoxifen-treated group, 1.3% vs 0.4%, and two patients in the tamoxifen-treated group died of pulmonary emboli.

There was an increased incidence of endometrial carcinoma in women who were randomized to receive tamoxifen. There were 21 endometrial carcinomas that occurred as first events in the tamoxifen-treated population (1.5%) compared with three in the placebo group. The estimated annual incidence of endometrial carcinoma was 1.9/1,000 women. The incidence of other second primary tumors, excluding endometrial cancers, was not significantly different in the two groups.

Hot flashes, vaginal discharge, and irregular menses were more frequent in women who were treated with tamoxifen

Five Years of Tamoxifen vs Ten Years of Tamoxifen (Second Randomization)

The average time on study for this "second randomization" was 48 months. All study treatment was terminated in December of 1995 when it became apparent that there was no additional advantage associated with prolonging the administration of tamoxifen beyond 5 years. Thus, for the second randomization, patients assigned to additional tamoxifen received an average of 4 additional years (9 years in total) instead of the protocol-mandated period of 5 years (10 years in total). Data from the 1,153 eligible patients indicated that there was a significant disease-free survival advantage in favor of patients who stopped tamoxifen after 5 years compared to those randomized to receive 10 years of tamoxifen, 92% vs 86% (*P* = 0.003, Table 2). Distant disease-free survival differences were similarly in favor of the 5 year group compared to 10 years of tamoxifen, 96% vs 90% (*P* = 0.01). Although the survival differences only approached statistical significance, they, too, favored the group that stopped tamoxifen at 5 years, with overall survival being 96% for the 5-year group and 94% for the group randomized to 10 years (*P* = 0.08).

Table 2

Second Randomization: 5 Years of Tamoxifen vs 10 Years

	5 Yrs Tam	10 Yrs Tam	P
DFS	92%	86%	0.003
DDFS	96%	90%	0.01
S	96%	94%	0.08

Tam = tamoxifen, DFS = disease-free survival, DDFS = distant disease-free survival, S = survival.

These differences were also reflected in a greater number of events occurring in the group randomized to 10 years of tamoxifen, 66 vs 36. These events were not limited to non-life-threatening sites, in that there was an increased number of distant failures in the group randomized to 10 years of tamoxifen, 16 vs 7. For the patients in the second randomization, there continued to be an increased number of endometrial cancers in the group receiving 10 years of tamoxifen. Although the numbers are small, here were 6 endometrial carcinomas in the group receiving 10 years of tamoxifen compared to 3 in those receiving 5 years of tamoxifen. Moreover, there did not appear to be a continued benefit in the reduction of ipsilateral breast cancer occurrence following 5 years of treatment and this lack of further benefit appeared true for the contralateral breast as well. Deaths without evidence of disease were not reduced in the 10-year tamoxifen cohort: There were 9 such deaths in the 10-year group compared to 5 in patients receiving 5 years of tamoxifen. This information is relevant when assessing the potential reduction in fatal cardiac events attributable to prolonged tamoxifen administration.

Thus, there is clearly no advantage to prolonging tamoxifen beyond 5 years; if anything, there is a small but significant dimunition in disease-free survival and distant disease-free survival. In the second randomization, as was the case in the first randomization, there were no differences related to age, in that results in women younger than 50 years of age and women older than 49 years were similar. Other characteristics, such as tumor size and progesterone receptors, showed no interaction with duration of tamoxifen treatment.

Commentary

It is essential that conclusions based on results from protocol B-14 be kept in perspective. Although, clearly, 10 years of tamoxifen is not superior to 5 years, this finding should not be confused with the overall observation derived from the initial and principal randomization. When tamoxifen is compared to placebo (eg, those patients who never received tamoxifen), there continues to be a highly significant benefit in disease-free survival, distant disease-free survival, and overall survival in favor of tamoxifen. The data are incontrovertible in confirming that tamoxifen is a highly effective and relatively non-toxic therapy in women with stage I breast cancer.

A great deal has been written in the past several years about the increased incidence of endometrial carcinoma associated with tamoxifen. The estimated annual incidence of endometrial carcinoma in this patient cohort was 1.9 per 1,000 women. This is certainly no greater than the incidence of endometrial carcinoma associated with the use of estrogen replacement therapy in postmenopausal women. While the increased incidence of endometrial carcinoma associated with tamoxifen must be viewed with utmost concern, it seems inexplicable that estrogen replacement therapy is prescribed in a seemingly perfunctory manner in healthy patients, whereas a similar risk of endometrial cancer associated with tamoxifen has resulted in a host of regulatory interventions both in the treatment of women with breast cancer, as well as in those women at high risk for developing breast cancer who are participating in tamoxifen-related prevention trials.

The data are incontrovertible in confirming that tamoxifen is a highly effective and relatively non-toxic therapy in women with stage I breast cancer

One of the most important and often overlooked benefits associated with tamoxifen is the dramatic reduction in the incidence of ipsilateral breast tumor recurrence in those women treated with breast-preserving operations and postoperative radiotherapy. The three-fold reduction in ipsilateral breast tumor recurrence is of considerable relevance relative to quality of life and the cost of health care delivery. The rationale for a breast-preserving operation is obviously to preserve the breast; at 10 years, 10% of the placebo group developed a local breast tumor recurrence compared to 3.4% in the tamoxifen group. Women who developed a tumor recurrence in the ipsilateral breast were generally treated with a mastectomy, a therapeutic convention that is still very much applied today. Since breast-preserving procedures are being performed with greater frequency, the number of patients who are able to preserve their breast as a result of tamoxifen therapy is cumulatively increasing. Because ipsilateral breast tumor recurrences were included as events in the analysis of disease-free survival, and since only 38% of the initial patient population (principal randomization) was treated with breast preserving operations, the benefits in disease-free survival for the overall population tend to underestimate the results that would have been achieved in a population limited to patients treated with lumpectomy.

At the initiation of the principal randomization in early 1982, it was thought that tamoxifen might prolong survival by reducing fatal cardiac events. It is still contended by some that the utility of tamoxifen in the adjuvant setting cannot be measured simply by its effects in controlling breast cancer recurrence, but potential reduction in cardiac events, osteoporosis and major fractures, the potential delay in the onset of organic brain syndrome, must also be taken into account when assessing the overall benefit of this agent.

It has become abundantly clear that such ancillary end points, at least in the stage I breast cancer setting, will not influence outcome. It has become equally clear that the breast cancer setting is not the appropriate model in which to determine the cardiac and bone effects of tamoxifen. There was no reduction in the overall number of patients dying without evidence of disease in patients treated with prolonged tamoxifen and it would have been in this cohort that any potential reduction in fatal cardiac events would have been detected. These ancillary endpoints are, however, being addressed in the current Breast Cancer Prevention Trial (BCPT), NSABP protocol P-1, where women at high risk for the development of breast cancer are randomized to receive a placebo or 5 years of tamoxifen treatment.

The fact that women < 50 years of age, those thought for many years not to be responsive to tamoxifen, demonstrate at least the same benefit as women older than 49 should probably stimulate a reassessment of the use of tamoxifen together with chemotherapy in women with histologically positive nodes. It would be surprising, although certainly not impossible, that women with histologically positive nodes would demonstrate a different response to tamoxifen by age when it has been clearly shown that women with node-negative disease benefit uniformly, regardless of age.

The results obtained with the "second randomization where patients receiving 5 years of tamoxifen were compared with those who were randomized to receive 10 years of tamoxifen are as counterintuitive as they are perplexing. The arduous quest to determine the optimal duration of tamoxifen administration has been punctuated by a number of phases; the preliminary trials initiated in the 1970s disclosed a cautious and circumspective approach exemplified by tamoxifen being given for 1 or 2 years. In keeping with the belief that tamoxifen was cytostatic and in light of preliminary demonstrations that 3 years were better than 2 years of tamoxifen, a more cavalier approach began to emerge; many serious and well informed clinical investigators believed that tamoxifen should be given indefinitely. The data from the 5- vs 10-year second randomization has certainly brought this era to a convincing and abrupt halt.

Although these findings are limited to patients with histologically negative nodes, the results from this study still provide the most compelling biological information relative to duration of treatment. While it is recognized that it is not justifiable to reflexly transpose this information to women with histologically positive nodes, it is apparent that the proponents of giving tamoxifen beyond 5 years to women with histologically positive nodes are now compelled to demonstrate that such an approach has merit using controlled clinical trials. Until such a demonstration is forthcoming, the NSABP has limited tamoxifen therapy in all its protocols, node negative and node positive, to a period of 5 years. The findings from a trial carried out by the Scottish Cancer Trials Breast Group[8], where patients who were free of disease after 5 years of tamoxifen treatment were re-randomized to no additional therapy or prolonged tamoxifen, also demonstrated that treatment beyond 5 years did not improve upon the results obtained at 5 years. Although the number of patients in this study is small, 173 patients on prolonged tamoxifen, 169 receiving 5 years, approximately 25% were node positive; there appeared to be no interaction between duration of treatment and nodal status.

The arduous quest to determine the optimal duration of tamoxifen administration has been punctuated by a number of phases

Not only do patients who receive more than 5 years of tamoxifen (an average of 9 years) not fare better than patients receiving 5 years of tamoxifen, but they actually have a significantly decreased disease-free survival and distant disease-free survival. This finding should lead to a number of new hypotheses that could be tested in the pre-clinical setting. Numerous theories have been promulgated to explain the seemingly detrimental effect of prolonging tamoxifen beyond 5 years in patients with histologically negative nodes. The most prevalent hypothesis suggests that long-term tamoxifen administration results in the development of resistance in persistent micrometastatic foci. This, of course, would not explain an increased incidence of breast tumor recurrence in the group receiving tamoxifen for longer duration.

A second and more plausible hypothesis suggests that after a given period of time, tamoxifen functions as an agonist and stimulates residual foci of micrometastatic disease. Whereas this hypothesis would explain the increased failure rate in the group randomized to receive 10 years of treatment, there are some findings from these analyses that are not immediately supportive of the agonist thesis. The annual failure rate per 1000 patients in the principal randomization was 56.6 for placebo and 37.6 for tamoxifen, with a mean time on study of 10 years; the rates at 5 years were similar. The group receiving prolonged tamoxifen in the second randomization seemed to have an identical annual failure rate compared to those patients randomized to tamoxifen in the initial randomization, namely 35.4. Although this represents an indirect comparison, there appears to be no evidence of a stimulatory effect when tamoxifen is prolonged beyond 5 years. The dramatic difference seems to be derived from those women who stopped the tamoxifen after 5 years where the annual failure rate per 1,000 patients fell to 19.3. It has been suggested, therefore, that the withdrawal of tamoxifen has an inhibitory effect that may not be related to an agonist phenomenon. Based on these findings, one might postulate that the administration of tamoxifen on an intermittent schedule should be seriously explored. Regardless of the hypothetical mechanism of action, however, the findings are unequivocal; an important question has been answered relative to the most commonly used therapeutic intervention in the management of primary breast cancer: tamoxifen should not be given beyond 5 years for women with node-negative disease.

References

1. NSABP halts B-14 trial: No benefit seen beyond 5 years of tamoxifen use. *J Natl Cancer Inst* 87:1829, 1995.

2. Fisher B, Redmond C, Brown A., et al: Adjuvant chemotherapy with and without tamoxifen in the treatment of primary breast cancer: Five-year results from the NSABP trial. *J Clin Oncol* 4:459-471, 1986.

3. Fisher B, Brown A., Wolmark N, et al: Prolonged tamoxifen therapy for primary breast cancer. Findings from an NSABP clinical trial. *Ann Intern Med* 106: 649-654, 1987.

4. Fisher B, Redmond C, Legault-Poisson S, et al: Postoperative chemotherapy and tamoxifen compared with tamoxifen alone in the treatment of positive-node breast cancer patients aged 50 years and older with tumors responsive to tamoxifen: Results from the National Surgical Adjuvant Breast and Bowel Project B-16. *J Clin Oncol* 8: 1005-1018, 1990.

5. Fisher B, Redmond C, Dimitrov NV, et al: A randomized clinical trial evaluating sequential methotrexate and fluorouracil in the treatment of patients with node-negative breast cancer who have estrogen receptor-negative tumors. *N Engl J Med* 320: 473-478, 1989.

6. Fisher B, Dignam J, Bryant J. et al: The worth of 5 versus more than 5 years of tamoxifen therapy for breast cancer patients with negative nodes and estrogen receptor positive tumors: An update of NSABP B-14. *JNCI* 88:1529-1542, 1996.

7. Fisher B, Costantino J, Redmond C, et al: A randomized clinical trial evaluating tamoxifen in the treatment of patients with node-negative breast cancer who have estrogen receptor-positive tumors. *N Engl J Med* 320: 479- 484, 1989.

8. Scottish Cancer Trials Breast Group, Edinburgh: Randomised comparison of five years of adjuvant tamoxifen with continuous therapy for operable breast cancer. *Br J Cancer* 74:297-299, 1996.

Chapter 9

Endometrial Cancer and Tamoxifen

Richard R. Barakat, MD
Assistant Attending Surgeon
Gynecology Service
Memorial Sloan-Kettering Cancer Center

Tamoxifen, a nonsteroidal antiestrogen, was first approved by the US Food and Drug Administration for the treatment of patients with breast cancer in 1978. Large clinical trials involving over 75,000 patients have demonstrated an improved recurrence-free and overall survival benefit in both pre- and postmenopausal women. Long-term adjuvant tamoxifen is the hormonal treatment of choice for selected patients with breast cancer, and large-scale trials are currently underway to evaluate its role as a chemopreventative agent in healthy women at risk for breast cancer.

One of the most significant potential complications of long-term tamoxifen use is the development of endometrial cancer. Tamoxifen is believed to exert its main effect by blocking the binding of estrogen to the estrogen receptor. Although primarily an antiestrogen, tamoxifen also exhibits some mild estrogenic actions. Following the initial report by Killackey[1] suggesting a possible link between tamoxifen use and the development of endometrial carcinoma in three patients, approximately 250 additional cases of tamoxifen-associated uterine cancer have been reported.[2] Recently, the results of the National Surgical Adjuvant Breast and Bowel Project (NSABP) B-14 trial were published.[3] This randomized trial of tamoxifen vs placebo in women with estrogen -receptor-positive breast cancer confined to the breast with negative axillary nodes revealed a 7.5-fold increase in the risk of developing endometrial cancer in the tamoxifen-treated group.

The indications for tamoxifen use have broadened to include long-term adjuvant therapy as well as preventative therapy for selected high-risk women. Consequently, a large number of individuals, including healthy young women with no history of cancer, will be subjected to the long-term effects of tamoxifen. The purpose of this chapter is to review the current literature regarding endometrial cancer in breast cancer patients being treated with tamoxifen, and to explore the role of screening for endometerial cancer in these patients.

Endometrial Cancer and Tamoxifen

Despite the overwhelming benefit of tamoxifen for prevention of breast cancer recurrence, many patients worry about the possibility of developing endometrial cancer. Risk of developing endometrial cancer among tamoxifen-treated patients has been defined by results of the NSABP trial B-14. Data on the rates of endometrial and other cancers were analyzed for 2,843 patients with node-negative, ER-positive, invasive breast cancer randomly assigned to placebo or tamoxifen (20 mg/day) as well as for 1,220 tamoxifen-treated patients registered on NSABP B-14 subsequent to randomization. Two of the 1,424 patients assigned to receive placebo developed endometrial cancer; both of these patients, however, had subsequently received tamoxifen for treatment of breast cancer recurrence. Fifteen patients randomized to tamoxifen treatment developed endometrial cancer, although one of these patients never actually accepted therapy. Eight additional cases of uterine cancer occurred among the 1,220 tamoxifen-treated patients, 76% of which were in women 60 years of age or older. The mean duration on tamoxifen therapy was 35 months. Thirty-six percent of the endometrial cancers developed within 2 years of beginning therapy and six cases occurred fewer than 9 months after treatment was initiated, suggesting that some of the cancers may have been present prior to starting tamoxifen therapy.

The average annual risk of developing endometrial cancer in the placebo group was 0.2/1,000 compared with 1.6/1,000 for the randomized tamoxifen-treated group. This is an important figure that clinicians may pass on to their patients. Physicians should counsel patients on tamoxifen that their annual risk of developing endometrial cancer is approximately 2/1,000 or 0.2%. Furthermore, any discussion regarding the risk of endometrial cancer with tamoxifen treatment must also take into account the benefits of tamoxifen with respect to reducing both breast cancer recurrence and new contralateral breast cancers. In the B-14 trial, the cumulative rate/1,000 of breast cancer relapse was 227.8 in the placebo group compared to 123.5 in the tamoxifen-treated group. In addition, the cumulative rate of contralateral breast cancer was reduced from 40.5 to 23.5, respectively, in the two groups. Even taking into account the increased cumulative rate of endometrial cancer, there was a 38% reduction in the 5-year cumulative risk of cancer recurrence in the tamoxifen-treated group. Many patients are reassured by these data.

The Role of Screening

Published data would appear to support an association between tamoxifen and the development of both benign and malignant endometrial neoplasia. The increased risk of endometrial cancer associated with tamoxifen use increases morbidity in breast cancer patients but does not appear to outweigh the significant advantage that tamoxifen confers by controlling breast cancer. This issue is clear for the patient with a diagnosis of breast cancer. Of greater concern, however, are the implications for healthy, albeit high-risk, women considering tamoxifen because of family histories of breast cancer. Large-scale trials of tamoxifen as a chemopreventative agent are now underway in England and the US. Whether the postulated reduction in breast cancer outweighs the risk of endometrial cancer in this population remains to be determined.

Large-scale trials of tamoxifen as a chemopreventative agent are now underway in England and the US

Endometrial Biopsy

What, if any, recommendations can be made at this point regarding screening for endometrial cancer in breast cancer patients on tamoxifen? First, the expected annual risk of endometrial cancer is approximately 2/1,000, as defined by the B-14 trial. A screening program may detect premalignant endometrial precursors such as atypical hyperplasia or benign endometrial conditions including polyps, the incidence of which will be higher than 2/1,000.

The best method for screening, however, remains to be determined. Some have proposed annual endometrial sampling, although this is not without its difficulties. In one study, investigators were unable to perform office endometrial biopsies with a Novak curette in 44% of 89 postmenopausal patients due to atrophic changes.[4] Clinicians who recommend office endometrial biopsies to their patients must be prepared for the possibility of being unable to access the endometrial cavity. Should these patients then be subjected to the inherent morbidity of a fractional dilatation and curettage (D&C) under general anesthesia? Barakat et al[5] presented the preliminary results of a prospective endometrial screening study in tamoxifen-treated breast cancer patients at the 1995 Annual Meeting of the American Society of Clinical Oncology. One hundred twenty-six patients with a mean age of 51 years were entered on the study; six (4.8%) could not undergo the biopsy procedure due to a stenotic cervix. Of the remaining 120 patients, 7 (5.8%) were noncompliant, 4 were removed from the study due to progression of breast cancer, 4 discontinued use of tamoxifen, and 4 were considered protocol violations. The remaining 101 evaluable patients underwent a total of 296 biopsies (mean, 3), utilizing a Pipelle endometrial biopsy device (Unimar; Wilmington, Conn.), with a median surveillance time of 16.2 months. Four (4%) biopsies were abnormal, including two complex hyperplasias, one atypical hyperplasia, and one with an abnormal amount of histiocytes. All abnormal biopsies were confirmed by fractional D&C. Six (6%) additional patients required D&C for persistent bleeding despite benign biopsies. The findings at D&C included polyps (3), benign endometrium (2), and pseudodecidualization (a benign effect due to progesterone therapy) in one patient. Three patients underwent hysterectomy. The first developed complex atypical hyperplasia following 12 months of tamoxifen. The second underwent a hysterectomy for a pelvic mass—which, on final pathology, revealed a high-grade leiomyosarcoma—following 15 months of tamoxifen. A third patient underwent hysterectomy for complex hyperplasia with extensive mucinous change after 13 months of tamoxifen. The authors concluded that office endometrial biopsies can be used to monitor the endometrium in the majority (95%) of breast cancer patients on tamoxifen. Six percent of patients may require a D&C for persistent bleeding. Significant pathology was detected by endometrial biopsy in two (2%) patients, and by close surveillance in a third. However, longer follow-up will be required to determine the value of routine endometrial biopsies in tamoxifen-treated breast cancer patients.

Transvaginal Sonography

Transvaginal sonography may provide a non-invasive means of screening for endometrial pathology in tamoxifen-treated breast cancer patients. The definition of an abnormal endometrial stripe remains to be defined. As reported by Lahti et al[6], if a cutoff of > 5 mm was used to define an abnormal endometrial echo, 22 (51.2%) patients had no abnormal endometrial pathology. Kedar et al[7] reported a predictive value of 100% (16/16) for atypical hyperplasia or polyps with an endometrial stripe of > 8 mm. These findings suggest that premalignant changes can be detected with transvaginal sonography and that the use of ultrasound and/or endometrial sampling to screen for endometrial neoplasia needs to be evaluated in large prospective trials before recommendations for screening can be made.

Care must be taken, however, to avoid over-interpretation of ultrasonographic findings of the endometrium in tamoxifen-treated patients. Goldstein[8] recently reported five postmenopausal tamoxifen-treated patients who, on routine surveillance with vaginal probe ultrasonography, were described as having heterogeneous, bizarre-appearing endometria with multiple sonolucent areas suggestive of a polyp. Because of concerns regarding tamoxifen use and endometrial neoplasia, the first patient was referred for a curettage and hysteroscopy. Minimal tissue was obtained and hysteroscopic evaluation revealed a smooth atrophic endometrium. When the abnormal sonographic appearance persisted, the patient underwent a sonohysterogram, which involves the instillation of 3 to 10 mL of saline at the time of sonography. The fluid enhancement revealed that the changes originally interpreted as endometrial were actually subendometrial in origin. Four additional patients with similar abnormal sonographic findings were actually found to have subendometrial abnormalities on sonohysterogram. It is unclear what these abnormal areas represent as none of the patients have undergone hysterectomy. Some have speculated that they may represent adenomyomatous-like changes. Further studies regarding the sonographic appearance of the endometrium in tamoxifen-treated patients are warranted.

Screening Issues

Many patients with breast cancer who are taking tamoxifen worry a great deal about the possibility of developing a different cancer. Clinicians who care for these patients sense this anxiety and, in an effort to help may attempt to screen for endometrial cancer. Although the chance of detecting endometrial cancer is very low, the patient may benefit from the reassurance that a negative test provides. The ultimate goal of any screening study is to detect cancer at an earlier stage and thereby improve outcome. To date, there is no evidence that any form of screening for endometrial cancer in tamoxifen-treated patients will accomplish this.

First, the majority of tamoxifen-associated endometrial cancers appear to be have a similar stage, grade, histology, and prognosis as endometrial cancers occurring in the general population.[9] Since their prognosis is generally good, early detection will probably not improve outcome. Furthermore, the treatment for preinvasive cancer (atypical endometrial hyperplasia) is still hysterectomy; therefore, the patient will not gain any benefit by undergoing a less radical procedure. Approximately 80,000 of the 182,000

Table I

Recommendations for Women Taking Tamoxifen

• Annual gynecologic examination including Pap smear, bimanual and rectovaginal examination

• Patient counseling regarding the risk of endometrial cancer and reporting of symptoms (bloody discharge, spotting, abnormal bleeding)

• Prompt endometrial sampling for any abnormal bleeding

• Dilatation and curettage for biopsy which reveals endometrial hyperplasia to rule out a more significant lesion

• If tamoxifen must be continued, hysterectomy should be considered for atypical hyperplasia

• Tamoxifen can be continued following hysterectomy for atypical hyperplasia or carcinoma following discussion with the physician responsible for the patient's breast care women diagnosed with breast cancer annually will be started on tamoxifen. In addition, approximately 500,000 women are currently on tamoxifen. If one were to assume a 30% prior hysterectomy rate, this would leave 30% of 580,000, or 406,000 women, at risk for endometrial cancer by the end of the year. If the annual risk of developing endometrial cancer, according to the B-14 trial, is 2/1,000, this would result in approximately 812 cases (2/1,000 · 406,000) of endometrial cancer. A review of the published cases of tamoxifen-associated endometrial cancers revealed that approximately 15% of these patients will actually die from endometrial cancer.[10] If screening were able to detect endometrial cancer earlier and thus prevent deaths, potentially 15% of these 812 cases, or 122 deaths, could potentially be prevented—if one assumes a 100% efficacy for the screening method used. The cost of screening 406,000 women with either endometrial biopsy, transvaginal sonography, or both would, however, be extremely high.

Current Screening Recommendations

How then should clinicians follow their breast cancer patients on tamoxifen (Table 1)? According to a recent Committee Opinion of the American College of Obstetricians and Gynecologists (ACOG), women with breast cancer who take tamoxifen should undergo annual gynecologic evaluations, including Pap tests and pelvic exams.[11] Any abnormal bleeding, including bloody discharge, spotting, or other symptoms should be thoroughly evaluated by an endometrial biopsy. No distinction should be made based on the amount, color, or frequency of bleeding. In a review from Memorial Sloan-Kettering Cancer Center, Gibson et al[12] reported that all cases of endometrial carcinoma detected by D&C in tamoxifen-treated breast cancer patients presented with abnormal bleeding. ACOG further recommends that practitioners be alert to the increased incidence of endometrial malignancy, and screening procedures be employed at the discretion of the individual gynecologist. No comment, however, is made as to what these screening procedures should be. If atypical endometrial hyperplasia or carcinoma is detected, the patient should undergo a hysterectomy; however, tamoxifen can be reinstituted immediately afterwards. Although progestins are used to reduce the risk of endometrial hyperplasia and cancer in women on estrogen replacement, ACOG does not advocate this practice in breast cancer patients as the impact of progestins on the course of breast cancer is not known.

Perhaps the most important task that clinicians can perform is to educate and counsel their patients. All breast cancer patients taking tamoxifen need to know that the annual risk of endometrial cancer is 2/1,000. Furthermore, they should be informed that the majority of any cancers that develop have a low stage and grade, and are usually curable by hysterectomy. Moreover, they need to be informed that despite the increased risk of endometrial cancer, the overwhelming benefit is in favor of taking tamoxifen as shown by the results of the NSABP B-14 trial, which demonstrated a 38% reduction in the 5-year cumulative risk of cancer recurrence in the tamoxifen-treated group.

As more information is obtained about the effect of tamoxifen on the endometrium, and studies determine the sensitivity and specificity of various tests used to screen for endometrial cancer, more definite recommendations for following this group of patients can be made. For now, all women with breast cancer, whether or not they are receiving tamoxifen, should be encouraged to undergo annual gynecologic evaluation, which should include endometrial sampling in the presence of abnormal vaginal bleeding.

References

1. Killackey MA, Hakes TB, Pierce VK: Endometrial adenocarcinoma in breast cancer patients receiving antiestrogens. *Cancer Treat Rep* 69:237-238, 1985.

2. Assikis VJ, Jordan VC: Gynecologic effects of tamoxifen and the association with endometrial carcinoma. *Int J Gynecol Obstet* 49:241-257, 1995.

3. Fisher B, Costantino JP, Redmond CK, et al: Endometrial cancer in tamoxifen-treated breast cancer patients: Findings from the National Surgical Adjuvant Breast and Bowel Project (NSABP) B-14. *J Natl Cancer Inst* 86:527-537, 1994.

4. Gal D, Kopel S, Bashevkin M, et al: Oncologic potential of tamoxifen on endometria of postmenopausal women with breast cancer: Preliminary report. *Gynecol Oncol* 42:120-123, 1991.

5. Barakat RR, Gilewski TA, Saigo PE, et al: The effect of adjuvant tamoxifen on the endometrium in women with breast cancer: An interim analysis of a prospective study (abstract). *Proc Am Soc Clin Oncol* 779, 1995.

6. Lahti E, Blanco G, Kauppila A, et al: Endometrial changes in postmenopausal breast cancer patients receiving tamoxifen. *Obstet Gynecol* 81:660-664, 1993.

7. Kedar RP, Bourne TH, Powles TJ, et al: Effects of tamoxifen on uterus and ovaries of postmenopausal women in a randomised breast cancer prevention 13 trial. *Lancet* 343:1318-1321, 1994.

8. Goldstein SR: Unusual ultrasonographic appearance of the uterus in patients receiving tamoxifen. *Am J Obstet Gynecol* 170:447-451, 1994.

9. Barakat RR, Wong G, Curtin JP, et al: Tamoxifen use in breast cancer patients who subsequently develop corpus cancer is not associated with a higher incidence of adverse histologic features. *Gynecol Oncol* 55:164-168, 1994.

10. Barakat RR: The effect of tamoxifen on the endometrium. *Oncology* 9:129-139, 1995.

11. ACOG Committee Opinion: Tamoxifen and endometrial cancer. 169, 1996.

12. Gibson LE, Barakat RR, Venkatraman ES, et al: Endometrial pathology at dilatation and curettage in breast cancer patients: Comparison of tamoxifen users and nonusers. *Cancer J Sci Am* 2:35-38, 1996.

Chapter 10

Tamoxifen and Endometrial Cancer: The Worldwide Clinical Database

V. J. Assikis, MD
Research Fellow

V. Craig Jordan, PhD, DSc
Director, Breast Cancer Research Program
Robert H. Lurie Cancer Center
Northwestern University Medical School

The World Health Organization lists tamoxifen as an essential medicine for the treatment of breast cancer. However, in 1996 the International Agency for Research on Cancer declared tamoxifen to be a carcinogen based on laboratory studies in rats and the detection of endometrial cancers in women. Nevertheless, the Agency stated that their findings should not be used for regulatory purposes nor should any woman be denied tamoxifen based on concerns about the risks from the detection of endometrial cancer. The benefits of tamoxifen to aid the survival of patients with breast cancer exceed any risks.

In this chapter we will place the concerns about a link between tamoxifen and endometrial cancer in perspective. The key issue is the design of the studies conducted so far that have not prescreened women for endometrial cancer or have only screened tamoxifen-treated patients.

Endometrial Cancer Epidemiology

Endometrial cancer is the most common gynecologic malignancy. Estimates for 1996 project that 32,800 new cases will be diagnosed and 5,900 cancer deaths will occur. Women with elevated endogenous estrogens (early menarche, obesity, Stein-Leventhal syndrome, estrogen-secreting ovarian tumors) or exogenous unopposed estrogens (estrogen replacement therapy) are typically at increased risk for endometrial cancer. In this group of patients, the development of endometrial carcinoma is usually preceded by a benign precursor, endometrial hyperplasia, that slowly develops with increasing degrees of cytologic atypia over time. Typically, small segments of the tumor outgrow their blood supply during the early exophytic growth phase, resulting in focal necrosis, which, in turn, gives rise to the symptom of postmenopausal bleeding. These early symptoms prompt women to seek medical attention at a time when the tumor is usually still confined to the uterus. Indeed, the SEER data[1] show that the majority of endometrial cancers are of low stage (stage I = 74%) and the overall 5-year survival rates are high (83%).

There is, however, a minority of endometrial carcinomas that demonstrate a diferent clinical behavior. These tumors are of aggressive histologic types (serous carcinoma, papillary carcinoma, clear cell carcinoma) and usually occur in women who have endometrial atrophy and lack the risk factors described earlier for estrogen-dependent endometrial disease. In addition, although tumors of mesenchymal origin, namely sarcomas, comprise only a small percentage of uterine tumors, they exhibit quite aggressive clinical behavior. Typically, these tumors are associated with a history of pelvic radiation exposure, while there is evidence of a possible link with stimulation by high estrogen levels.

The mean age of patients diagnosed with endometrial cancer is 59 years, but age seems to play a role in the pattern of tumors detected. Elderly patients have an increased incidence of endometrial cancer and a tendency towards more virulent histologic types that result in invasive, aggressive disease.[2] The increased virulence of endometrial cancer in the elderly may be related to the tumors' independence from hormonal factors.

Tamoxifen and Endometrial Cancer

In the past decade there have been a number of reports regarding the interaction of tamoxifen with the female reproductive tract. While endometrial cancer has been the main focus, tamoxifen has also been associated with minor changes in gonadotrophin levels, amenorrhea and oligomenorrhea, ovarian hyperstimulation in premenopausal women occasionally leading to ovarian cysts, exacerbation or regression of endometriosis, promotion of the growth of uterine leiomyomas and endometrial polyps, and there are even isolated case reports of women who developed ovarian or fallopian tube tumors and had a history of tamoxifen intake.[3] In general, the gynecologic concerns are mainly anecdotal. Estrogenic effects of tamoxifen have been demonstrated in the vaginal epithelium and increased endometrial proliferation has been observed in about one third of treated postmenopausal women.[3] The major clinical problem, however, has been the inability to predict which women will respond to tamoxifen as an estrogen-like substance and which will not.

Since 1985, a number of reports linking tamoxifen to endometrial cancer have appeared in the world literature. Many of these cases represent non-controlled case reports and most were collected retrospectively. In addition, a number of double-blind randomized trials have documented an increased frequency of endometrial cancer in tamoxifen-treated patients. These trials, however, were not designed to specifically answer the question of an association between tamoxifen and endometrial cancer. A number of biases may thus confound the results of these studies.[4] In none of these trials did the patients have a baseline endometrial screening for any existing lesions before they started taking tamoxifen, nor were they randomized in respect to major risk factors for the development of endometrial cancer. It can, therefore, not be excluded that a significant number of these women already had an undetected endometrial malignancy. In support of this notion are the findings of a large series of autopsies that showed that the incidence of occult endometrial cancer was 5 times higher than the reported rate for the same geographical area and the same period of time.[5]

The benefits of tamoxifen on overall survival of patients with breast cancer exceed any risks

There are now more than 7 million woman-years of experience with tamoxifen treatment worldwide. Since uterine toxicity is the most prominent adverse effect associated with tamoxifen treatment, there has been intense interest in reporting cases regarding endometrial abnormalities, both benign and malignant. In the past decade a number of reports have linked tamoxifen with the detection of endometrial cancer. We have previously reviewed the literature and found a total of only 349 endometrial carcinomas reported in tamoxifen-treated patients (Table 1, next page).[3,4] A number of sarcomas and mixed Müllerian tumors (MMT) have also been reported in association with tamoxifen treatment and are listed separately. Contrary to recent concerns expressed in regard to the potentially detrimental endometrial effects of tamoxifen in premenopausal women,[6] the vast majority of the reported endometrial cancers have occurred in postmenopausal women. Although the duration of tamoxifen therapy is not reported for all cases, it appears that both short-term (≤ 2 years) and long-term therapy (> 2 years) are implicated in the higher frequency of endometrial tumors. The daily dose of tamoxifen administered to these patients varies among the different reports, with 20 mg as the prevailing dosage. Some investigators have suggested that doses higher than the current standard (20 mg/day) may lead to an increase in the detection of endometrial cancer, however, our database provides no clear-cut evidence of such a relationship.

Is Tamoxifen Related to a More Aggressive Endometrial Cancer?

In 1993, a case-control study from Yale was published in the *Journal of Clinical Oncology*.[7] The authors conducted a retrospective search of the Yale/New Haven tumor registry for the decade 1980-1990. After screening 3,457 records, they identified 53 breast cancer patients who later on developed a uterine tumor. Fifteen of these patients had a history of 40 mg/day of tamoxifen intake for an average of 4.2 years. Ten of these tumors (67%) were of aggressive histologic type (high-grade endometrioid carcinoma, MMT, clear cell carcinoma, papillary serous carcinoma) and one-third of the patients died of endometrial cancer. The authors concluded that ". . . women receiving tamoxifen are at risk for high-grade endometrial cancers that have a poor prognosis. . . ."

This report created a lot of concern among clinicians as it challenged the long-standing belief that endometrial tumors arising in tamoxifen-treated patients have a favorable outcome, as do endometrial tumors in patients with a history of estrogen replacement therapy (ERT).

To address this issue, we have gathered all the available data on stage and grade of endometrial carcinomas occurring in tamoxifen-treated patients.[4] Stage is reported for 234 of these patients and grade is reported for 225 of them. In Table 2 we have compared the stage of endometrial tumors as reported in the Yale study[7] with the data from our literature review[4] as well as the SEER data.[1] There is general agreement that endometrial cancer detected in tamoxifen-treated women is typically confined to the uterus. Comparing the same three data sources, we have depicted the data on grade in Figure 1. As the figure shows, there is significant discrepancy among the three data sources. Contrary to the Yale data, which showed a predominance of high-grade tumors, our review shows

Table 1

Detection and Distribution of Uterine Malignancies in Patients Exposed to Tamoxifen

Endometrial carcinomas	349
Mixed Müllerian Tumors	18
Sarcomas	9
Patients	
Postmenopausal	200
Premenopausal	2
Duration of tamoxifen therapy	
≤ 2 years	91
> 2 years	108

Information derived from Assikis et al[4] with permission.

Table 2

Distribution of the Stage of Endometrial Cancer in the Yale Study[7], a Review of the International Literature[4] and the SEER Database[1]

	Yale		Review		SEER
Stage I	7/9	78%	184/234	79%	74%
Stage II-IV	2/9	22%	50/234	21%	26%

that, similar to the SEER data, endometrial cancer in patients treated with tamoxifen is of low (grade 1) or intermediate (grade 2) grade. Indeed, no other clinical study supports the Yale study.

Endometrial Cancer and the Duration of Tamoxifen

The first large-scale prospective clinical trial that offered evidence of a possible association between tamoxifen and endometrial cancer was the Stockholm trial.[8] A total of 1,846 patients were randomized to receive either

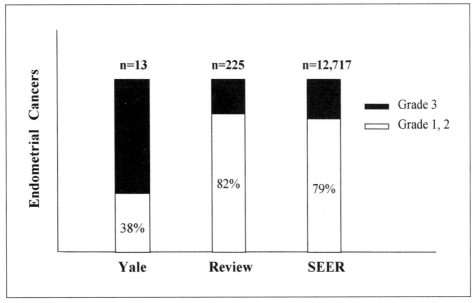

FIGURE I

40 mg of tamoxifen or placebo for 2 years. Patients who were initially random-ized to take tamoxifen for 2 years were offered the option to be re-randomized to receive tamoxifen for another 3 years, for a total of 5 years. Although tamoxifen proved beneficial in controlling second primary breast cancer, there was an increase in the incidence of endometrial cancer. This increase was reported to be higher for the long-term tamoxifen therapy (> 2 years) group than the short-term (≤ 2 years) group and led the authors to conclude that ". . . the cumulative frequency of endometrial cancers was significantly greater in patients who continued on tamoxifen than in those who stopped at 2 years. . . ." Four years later, the same group published an update of their findings, containing the individual characteristics of all the patients afflicted with endometrial cancer.[9] Seventeen endometrial cancers were diagnosed in the tamoxifen-treated group and five in the control group.

Interestingly, plotting the actual data (Figure 2) leads to a conclusion different than the one reported by the Stockholm group. It is apparent from Figure 2 that the majority of endometrial cancer cases (13/17) occurred in patients who had been treated with tamoxifen for 2 years or less.[10]

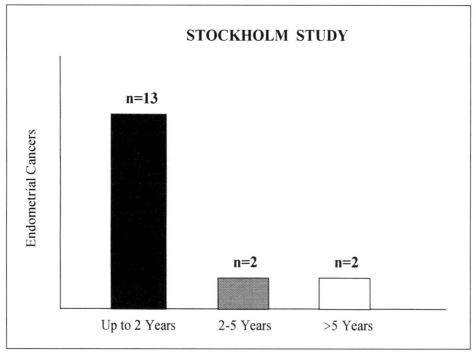

FIGURE 2

The results of the NSABP B-14 trial[11] showed that most tumors were of low grade and stage and that the rate of detection of endometrial cancer was constant over time on the drug. Interestingly, there are clinical trials, concerning both short-term (Christie Hospital trial) and long-term therapy (Scottish trial), that have failed to detect an increase in the frequency of endometrial cancer in association with tamoxifen treatment.[3] With the thousands of women having taken or currently receiving tamoxifen, there would have been an "epidemic" of endometrial malignancies by now should the effect of tamoxifen be as detrimental to the endometrium as some investigators have suggested.[12] Clearly, this is not the case. Based on the findings of the world's literature and those of randomized clinical trials, we believe that tamoxifen treatment confers a two- to three-fold increase in the detection of pre-existing endometrial cancer.[3,11]

It is imperative that patients with breast cancer are not denied the benefits of tamoxifen

Conclusions

The development of tamoxifen is one of the few success stories in the treatment of breast cancer. The drug is now the adjuvant treatment of choice for all stages of hormonal-responsive breast cancer. Its success as an antineoplastic agent has much to do with its low toxicity profile, despite the fact that the most significant side effect has been a modest increase in the detection of endometrial malignancies. Estrogenic properties of the drug are believed to account for this growth-promoting effect on the uterus, but current evidence suggests that tamoxifen's effect on the uterine tissues is more complicated than those typically seen with ERT.[13,14]

In the past decade a great number of investigators have looked into the association of tamoxifen with endometrial growth. Although the exact mechanisms by which tamoxifen exerts its growth-promoting effects in some patients and growth-inhibiting effects in others are yet to be identified, there is evidence of an association between tamoxifen therapy and an increase in the detection of endometrial malignancies. The existing findings point more towards a stimulation of an already initiated uncontrolled endometrial growth rather than a carcinogenic insult. In support of this notion is the fact that no DNA adducts have been reported from human uterine samples.[15]

We have reviewed the world's literature and found that endometrial cancer detected in tamoxifen-treated women is not an aggressive malignancy but usually produces symptoms at early stages and can, therefore, be dealt with quite effectively. Taking into account the frequency of endometrial cancer reported in prospective trials, in conjunction with the findings of case-control studies, we conclude that tamoxifen produces a 2/1,000 woman-years annual relative risk for endometrial cancer. The concern is mainly confined to post-menopausal women, and the dose of the drug does not seem to play a role.

Tamoxifen's benefit in the treatment of all stages of breast cancer is proven. It has been shown to prolong disease-free and overall survival, while maintaining a uniquely low toxicity profile.[16] Aggressive screening of tamoxifen-treated women carries the risk of identifying patients with benign endometrial changes that might alarm patients and clinicians but cannot be justified on the basis of cost-effectiveness. It is of utmost importance that physicians taking care of tamoxifen-treated women are well aware of these effects and do not consider stopping tamoxifen prematurely out of fear of an overestimated risk of secondary malignancies. The choice of monitoring techniques aiming to detect as early as possible any potential gynecological pathology is discussed in the preceding chapter and will not be addressed here. The benefits of tamoxifen in the treatment of breast cancer far outweigh any adverse gynecological effects. It is imperative that patients with breast cancer are not denied the benefits of tamoxifen. The risk of dying from endometrial cancer is far less than the risk of dying from recurrence of breast cancer.

References

1. National Cancer Institute: SEER Cancer Statistics Review 1973-1990, Document 932789. Bethesda, NM:NCI, 1993.

2. Hoffman K, Nekhlyudov L, Deligdisch L: Endometrial carcinoma in elderly women. *Gynecol Oncol* 58:198-201, 1995.

3. Assikis VJ, Jordan VC: Gynecologic effects of tamoxifen and the association with endometrial carcinoma. *Int J Gynecol Obstet* 49:241-257, 1995.

4. Assikis VJ, Neven P, Jordan VC, et al: A realistic clinical perspective of tamoxifen and endometrial carcinogenests. *Eur J Cancer* 32A:1464-1476, 1996.

5. Horwitz RI, Feinstein AR, Horwitz SM, et al: Necropsy diagnosis of endometrial cancer and detection-bias in case/control studies. *Lancet* 2:66–68, 1981.

6. Sasco AJ: Tamoxifen and menopausal status: Risks and benefits. *Lancet* 347:761, 1996.

7. Magriples U, Naftolin F, Schwartz PE, et al: High-grade endometrial carcinoma in tamoxifen-treated breast cancer patients. *J Clin Oncol* 11:485-490, 1993.

8. Fornander T, Rutqvist LE, Cedermark B, et al: Adjuvant tamoxifen in early breast cancer: Occurrence of new primary cancers. *Lancet* 1:117-120, 1989.

9. Fornander T, Helistrom AC, Moberger B: Descriptive clinicopathologic study of 17 patients with endometrial cancer during or after adjuvant tamoxifen in early breast cancer. *J Natl Cancer Inst* 85:1850-1855, 1993.

10. Jordan VC, Morrow M: Should clinicians be concerned about the carcinogenic potential of tamoxifen? *B Eur J Cancer* 30A:1714-1721, 1994.

11. Fisher B, Costantino JP, Redmond CK, et al: Endometrial cancer in tamoxifen-treated breast cancer patients: Findings from the National Surgical Adjuvant Breast and Bowel Project (NSABP) B-14. *J Natl Cancer Inst* 186:527-537, 1994.

12. DeGregorio MW, Maenpaa JU, Wiebe VJ: Tamoxifen for the prevention of breast cancer: No, in DeVita VT, Heilman S, Rosenberg SA (eds): *Important Advances in Oncology.* Philadelphia, JB Lippincott, 1995.

13. Decensi A, Fontana V, Bruno S, et al: Effect of tamoxifen on endometrial proliferation. *J Clin Oncol* 14:434-440, 1996.

14. Goldstein SR: Unusual ultrasonographic appearance of the uterus in patients receiving tamoxifen. *Am J Obstet Gynecol* 170:447-451, 1994.

15. Carmichael PL, Ugwumadu AHN, Neven P, et al: Lack of genotoxicity of tamoxifen in human endometrium. *Cancer Res* 56:1475-1479, 1996.

16. Early Breast Cancer Trialists' Collaborative Group: Systemic treatment of early breast cancer by hormonal, cytotoxic, or immune therapy: 133 randomized trials involving 31000 recurrences and 24000 deaths in 75000 women. *Lancet* 339:1-15, 71-85, 1992.

Chapter 11

What To Do After Tamoxifen?

V. Craig Jordan, PhD, DSc
Director, Breast Cancer Research Program
Robert H. Lurie Cancer Center
Northwestern University Medical School

Tamoxifen is used for the treatment of breast cancer in pre- and post-menopausal women with all stages of breast cancer. However, tamoxifen may only be effective for a limited period of time and other treatment options must then be considered by the physician.

Resistance to tamoxifen therapy is complex and may occur at either the physiologic level or drug insensitivity may be a property of the tumor. Unfortunately, the molecular events of resistance to tamoxifen are imprecisely understood;[1] however, several general principles have emerged through the translation of laboratory concepts to clinical medicine.

In this chapter the potential forms of drug resistance will be considered and the rationale for the use of a therapeutic option will be presented. The concepts will be discussed in the form of a clinical scenario.

DRUG RESISTANCE

There are three potential mechanisms to explain the eventual failure of tamoxifen treatment:

1) Reversal of the effects of the antiestrogen with high estrogen levels.

2) Tamoxifen stimulated growth.

3) The loss of the estrogen receptor and the loss of hormone-dependent growth.

Reversal of the Effects of the Antiestrogen with High Estrogen Levels

Tamoxifen is an effective antitumor agent in premenopausal patients, however as pointed out in Chapter 6, tamoxifen can cause an increase in the circulatory levels of estrogens at all times in the menstrual cycle.[2] Estrogen levels can increase by 3 to 10 times, depending upon the time in the cycle when a comparison is made. Although the rise in estrogen may suggest that the antitumor actions of tamoxifen are being reversed, because it is a competitive inhibitor of estrogen action, there is no evidence that this occurs in the absence of clear cut information about disease recurrence. Indeed, it may be tempting to discontinue tamoxifen in the belief that the high level of circulating estrogen is a disadvantage to the patient, but there is no justification for the position that a premenopausal women will benefit without tamoxifen to block the action of her own estrogen in the tumor.

Clinical trials are currently evaluating the value of adjuvant tamoxifen with luteinizing-hormone-releasing-hormone superagonists, eg, goserelin (Zoladex). Goserelin is currently FDA approved and available as a treatment for the premenopausal patient with ER-positive advanced breast cancer.[3] It acts initially to hyperstimulate and ultimately to desensitize the pituitary gland from releasing the gonadotropins luteinizing and follicle-stimulating hormones that control steroidogenesis in the ovaries. Without gonadotropins the ovary becomes quiescent and stops producing estrogens (Figure 1). The

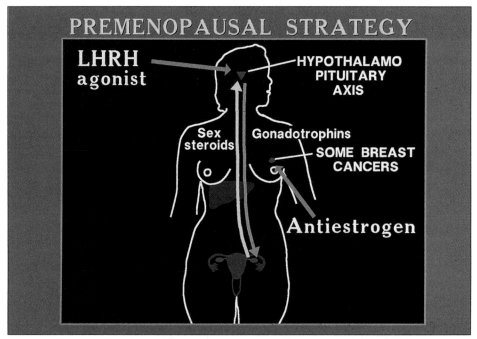

FIGURE I   Potential strategy for the treatment of the premenopausal patient with ER-positive breast cancer Tamoxifen is an acceptable therapeutic intervention despite an increase in circulating estradiol from the ovaries. Although tamoxifen is proven effective as an anti-breast-cancer agent, there is evidence that premenopausal patients who first respond to tamoxifen and then fail, can respond again to ovarian ablation. The LH-RH agonists are able to switch off the secretion of gonadotropins from the pituitary gland, which, in turn, stops ovarian steroidogenesis. The administration of sustained-release preparations of LH-RH superagonists represents a medical oophorectomy that is reversible once therapy is discontinued.

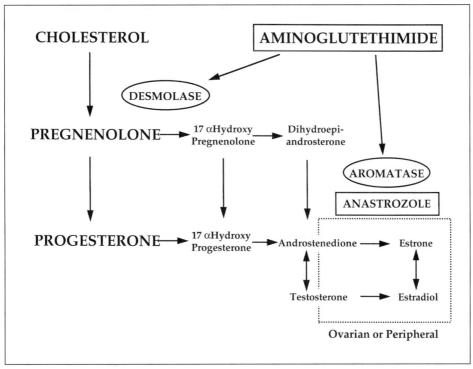

FIGURE 2   Aminoglutethimide exerts a dual action   It blocks the desmolase enzyme in the adrenal, as well as blocking peripheral aromatization enzyme systems. Anastrozole is targeted only to peripheral aromatase and is currently used for the treatment of advanced breast cancer after tamoxifen in postmenopausal women.

rapid fall in estrogen during the first month of treatment is equivalent to an oophorectomy, as the circulating estrogen levels are now in the postmenopausal range. However, the action of goserelin is reversible. The drug is administered as a once monthly subcutaneous injection of a sustained release formulation in a rice grain sized pellet. If the injections are discontinued, ovarian activity returns within 2 to 3 weeks.

Studies in premenopausal patients who receive tamoxifen to treat advanced breast cancer have shown that 30% to 50% of those who initially benefit from the antiestrogen can subsequently benefit from ovarian ablation following the failure of tamoxifen treatment. The inference is that tamoxifen can eventually be reversed by high circulating levels of estrogen in ER-positive disease, but only after tamoxifen is initially successful. The sustained release preparation of goserelin, Zoladex could be used as a medical oophorectomy in selected patients under these circumstances. Similarly the premenopausal

ER-positive, node-negative patient who has a recurrence after three to five years of adjuvant tamoxifen therapy could receive benefit from Zoladex when tamoxifen is stopped. The strategy is illustrated in Figure 1.

Tamoxifen Stimulated Growth

Laboratory studies using athymic mice have shown that long-term tamoxifen treatment can eventually cause the growth of ER-positive MCF-7 breast cancer cells into tumors. The cells are clonally selected so that either estrogen or tamoxifen can become the growth stimulus.[4] Tamoxifen-stimulated advanced breast cancer has been documented in postmenopausal patients who exhibit a withdrawal response when treatment is stopped.[5] However, tumor growth can become restimulated by the small, but adequate, levels of circulating estrogen in postmenopausal women.

Estrogen is made in postmenopausal women by the peripheral aromatization of the adrenal steroids androstenedione and testosterone (see Figure 2). Estrogen production is related to weight and is associated with the aromatase enzyme located in fatty tissue. Thus, non-estrogenic steroids secreted by the adrenals are converted to estradiol and estrone by peripheral aromatase enzyme systems and these estrogens ultimately activate the ER in metastatic breast cancers.

This knowledge provides an explanation for the success of adrenal ablation in the 1950s and 60s to treat postmenopausal patients with advanced breast cancer. However a chance observation with the drug aminoglutethimide, that was originally unsuccessfully used as an antiseizure medicine in children, showed that adrenal insufficiency occurred. Aminoglutethimide works in the adrenal by blocking the enzyme desmolase so all steroid synthesis stops. Regrettably, this action of aminoglutethimide also stops glucocorticoid synthesis that is essential for the ubiquitous control of metabolism. There is a feedback loop to the pituitary gland that ensures constant production of glucocorticoids through the pituitary hormone Adrenal Corticotropic Hormone (ACTH); if glucocorticoid levels fall, ACTH increases to cause more adrenal production of the appropriate steroids. Unfortunately the decrease in glucocorticoids produced by aminoglutethimide causes a reflex rise in pituitary ACTH that signals the adrenals to produce more steroids in general. Trials in breast cancer showed activity, but hydrocortisone has to be co-administered to maintain the drug's effectiveness.[6] The addition of hydrocortisone to the treatment with aminoglutethimide maintains a low level of ACTH and maintains the block on adrenal steroidogenesis.

Although an aminoglutethimide/hydrocortisone combination has been shown to be of value for the treatment of postmenopausal breast cancer, the toxicity and side effects of the therapy has precluded general use as a standard therapy. Fortunately aminoglutethmide also acts as an inhibitor of the peripheral aromatase enzyme system (see Figure 2). This provided the first clues that drugs could be targeted to the aromatase enzyme and avoid the adrenal target. This new strategy avoids the toxicities and complication of hydrocortisone coadministration.

The first specifically active aromatase enzyme blocker was 4-hydroxyandrostenedione, which acts as a suicide inhibitor of the enzyme. Drs. Harry and Angela Brodie first described the activities and antitumor properties of the compound at the Worcester Foundation for Experimental Biology in 1974-78.[7] Animal studies using the DMBA-induced rat mammary carcinoma model were started in 1974. They subsequently advocated clinical testing of the drug that is now approved and available for the treatment of advanced breast cancer in some countries. This discovery opened the door for the investigation of numerous more specific nonsteroidal compounds by the pharmaceutical industry. A range of drugs has been tested[8] but one compound, anastrozole (Arimidex) (Figure 3), is available in the United States for the treatment of ER-positive postmenopausal breast cancer after the failure of tamoxifen.[9] The principle is to deny a woman's own estrogen to the estrogen-receptor growth system by blocking synthesis of the hormone.

Another approach that is currently being explored is to develop com-

FIGURE 3 Compounds available as inhibitors of the aromatase enzyme system and for the treatment of postmenopausal women with advanced breast cancer.

pounds that block and destroy the ER in the tumor. Destruction of this essential transcription factor will prevent tumor cell replication and again deny estrogen access to its growth mechanism. The compounds should not exhibit any estrogen-like properties and will be like no estrogen at all.[10] These compounds, referred to as pure antiestrogens, were first described by Dr. Alan Wakeling at Zeneca Pharmaceuticals in the mid-1980s. The compounds inhibit tamoxifen-stimulated tumor growth in laboratory models of human breast and endometrial cancer and preliminary clinical trials in England have demonstrated activity in postmenopausal patients that eventually fail tamoxifen therapy.[12,13] No pure antiestrogens are currently available for general usage outside the context of a clinical trial.

The Loss of the ER and the Loss of Hormone Dependent Growth

Clinicians usually first exhaust the options of different endocrine therapies after a prolonged successful response to tamoxifen. However, the loss of the ER mechanism (determined by immunocytochemistry in a tissue biopsy) indicates only a low (< 10%) probability of a response to hormonal therapies. Nevertheless, combination chemotherapy with the most active agents can still produce objective long term responses in advanced breast cancer.

In summary, tamoxifen's proven effectiveness and established safety profile has made it the endocrine therapy of choice for all stages of breast cancer. Nevertheless, once successful treatment with tamoxifen is seen to fail, a range of other endocrine strategies is available to provide palliation for the patient with advanced disease before combination chemotherapy becomes the only option.

References

1. Tonetti D, Jordan VC: Possible mechanisms in the emergence of tamoxifen-resistant breast cancer. *Anticancer Drugs* 9:498-507, 1995.

2. Jordan VC, Fritz NF, Langan-Fahey S, et al: Alteration of endocrine parameters in premenopausal women with breast cancer during long-term adjuvant therapy with tamoxifen as a single agent. *J Natl Can Inst* 83:1488-1491, 1991.

3. Dixon AR, Jackson L, Nicholson RI, et al: The use of goserelin (Zoladex) in premenopausal advanced breast cancer. *Br J Cancer* 62:32, 1990

4. Gottardis MM, Jordan VC: Development of tamoxifen stimulated growth of MCF-7 tumors in athymic mice after long-term antiestrogen administration. *Cancer Res* 48:5183-5187, 1988.

5. Howell A, Dodwell DJ, Anderson H, et al: Response after withdrawal of tamoxifen and progestogens in advanced breast cancer. *Ann Oncol* 3:611-617, 1992.

6. Santen RJ, Manni A, Harvey, HA, et al: Endocrine treatment of breast cancer in women. *Endocrine Rev* 11:221-265, 1990.

7. Brodie AMH, Wing LY, Dowsett M, et al: Inhibitors of the aromatasse enzyme system: Basic and clinical studies with 4-hydroxyandrostenedione, in Jordan VC (ed): *Estrogen/Antiestrogen action and breast cancer therapy,* pp 221-234. Madison, University of Wisconsin Press, 1986.

8. Goss PE, Gwyn KMEH: Current perspectives on aromatase inhibitors in breast cancer. *J Clin Oncol* 12:2460-2470, 1994.

9. Plourde PV, Dyroff M, Dukes M: Arimidex: A potent and selective fourth generation aromatase inhibitor. *Breast Cancer Res Treat* 30:95-102, 1994.

10. Jordan VC: The only true antiestrogen is no estrogen. *Mol Cell Endocr* 74:91-95, 1990.

11. Wakeling AE: A new approach to breast cancer therapy—total estrogen ablation with pure antiestrogens, in Jordan VC (ed): *Long-Term Tamoxifen Treatment for Breast Cancer,* pp 219-234. University of Wisconsin Press, Madison, 1994.

12. Howell A, DeFriend D, Robertson J, et al: Response to a specific antioestrogen (ICI 182,780) in tamoxifen-resistant breast cancer. *Lancet* 345:29-30, 1995.

13. Howell A, DeFriend D, Robertson J, et al: Pharmacokinetics, pharmacological and antitumour efforts of the specific anti-oestrogen ICI 182, 780 in women with breast cancer. *Br J Cancer* 74:320-308, 1996.

Chapter 12

Talking With the Breast Cancer Patient About Tamoxifen

Amy S. Langer, MBA
Executive Director
National Alliance of Breast Cancer Organizations
(NABCO)

Communicating effectively with women about breast cancer—whether about risk, diagnosis or treatment—can be a challenge. This is both because the underlying issues are complex and because ongoing basic and clinical research continuously yields new and/or updated information. These two issues are particularly pertinent when the subject is tamoxifen, since this most widely prescribed oncology drug remains under extensive and ongoing investigation.

Despite the need to integrate new developments into clinical practice, certain basic issues and concerns are common to all discussions between breast cancer patients and health care providers when the subject is tamoxifen. At the National Alliance of Breast Cancer Organizations (NABCO), Information Services professionals have noted that tamoxifen is the single most common subject of inquiries received from breast cancer survivors. They also have found, however, that a handful of issues remain unclear to some women, and that certain necessary facts about the use of tamoxifen can be inadvertently overlooked.

What follows is an inventory of issues that should be covered as part of successful patient communications about tamoxifen—where a successful communication is defined as one in which the health care professional has offered a thorough and thoughtful review of needed information, and where the patient understands the issues, feels that her questions have been answered, and leaves the session confident that her plan of action is the appropriate one for her.

Why Use Tamoxifen?

The first and most important task of successful communication about tamoxifen is to explain the therapeutic rationale for use, whether it will be in the adjuvant setting or to control recurrent disease. It may also be appropriate to discuss why the drug may *not* be an option, since many women with breast cancer may already be aware of tamoxifen and wonder why it is not being prescribed.

A complete discussion on tamoxifen should include:

• The histology of the patient's tumor, its hormone receptor values, and other prognostic factors

• Results of studies on tamoxifen's benefits in this patient population, including quantitative assessments of reductions in recurrence risk and the risk of second breast cancers, or the probability of tamoxifen's ability to control breast cancer that has recurred

• How tamoxifen works

• How it will be administered, in what sequence, and for how long

• What systemic treatment alternatives to tamoxifen might also be considered, and their comparative benefits

• Additional benefits, still under study, that tamoxifen may confer in terms of cardiovascular health and osteoporosis, and how these benefits may vary in different patient groups (such as premenopausal women)

Given the importance of accruing breast cancer patients to clinical trials, the provider should consider whether the patient is eligible for any trials using tamoxifen. If so, the provider should conduct a detailed review of the trial's design and objectives, taking the patient through each section of the informed consent form.

Side Effects

After explaining the benefits of the drug, the next subject to be covered is an explanation of its risks. Although all medical interventions carry risks as well as benefits, the woman with breast cancer requires a realistic picture of how she should expect to feel while on the drug, and what risks she will be assuming in exchange for tamoxifen's benefits in controlling her disease.

Any discussion of tamoxifen must include a review of its most frequent side effects (such as hot flashes or vaginal symptoms), the potential severity of such symptoms, and at what point symptoms should be reported. Providers should also, of course, suggest ways to manage these uncomfortable side effects, both through lifestyle modifications (such as exercise, fluid intake, or layered clothing) and the use of specific products (such as vaginal lubricants).

Medical professionals understand the distinction between "minor" side effects or toxicities and "major" toxicities that may be life-threatening. Nevertheless, it is important to be aware that each patient has her own reactions and thresholds for side effects. Some women, particularly premenopausal women, may find that tamoxifen-related hot flashes are extremely disruptive of their work and family lives, to the extent that the acute distress associated with these symptoms overshadows longer-term concerns about breast cancer. These patients need attention and interventions.

It is also often useful to review the following:

- How tamoxifen might interact with other planned or current treatments for breast cancer, or with other types of medications (including anticoagulants)
- What to do if a pill is skipped or if the patient cannot recall whether she has taken it
- How to obtain educational materials on the drug's benefits and side effects, including the manufacturer's package insert; any questions that arise as a result of reading the package insert should be raised with the medical team.

All women on tamoxifen should obtain regular gynecological examinations, at least annually

[Many useful and often free resources are available to breast cancer patients for information and support (Table 1)].

Potentially Serious Risks

After reviewing potential side effects and management, the discussion should proceed to more serious risks. The risk of endometrial cancer in women who are taking tamoxifen is a subject that has received widespread media attention and needs to be thoroughly discussed and understood. Many women are not aware that a number of commonly prescribed drugs, including some forms of estrogen replacement therapy, have also been associated with secondary cancer risk—tamoxifen is by no means alone in this regard. And although it seems obvious, it can be useful to make clear that in hysterectomized women (a frequently performed procedure in the U.S.), risk of endometrial cancer is reduced to zero.

A discussion about the risks associated with tamoxifen treatment might also appropriately cover:

- The extent of endometrial and other cancer risks in women who have been diagnosed with breast cancer
- The extent to which tamoxifen's benefits in protecting against recurrent breast cancer or death from the disease vastly outweigh the small risk of endometrial cancer, which, when detected early, is curable
- Reports claiming that tamoxifen can cause other types of cancer, including liver cancer. The provider should explain that studies on this subject are ongoing, and that if indeed there is a risk, it is currently deemed to be not at all significant
- Information for premenopausal patients who might plan to become

Table I

Organizations for Breast Cancer Patients and Professionals

The American Cancer Society has voluntary programs concerned with breast cancer in its divisions and units nationwide. The ACS toll-free hot line, (800) ACS-2345, provides information on all forms of cancer, as well as referrals to the ACS-sponsored "Reach to Recovery" and "Look Good, Feel Better" programs. For more information, contact your local American Cancer Society office.

Cancer Care, Inc., based in New York City, is staffed by social work professionals offering support services, education and information, referrals and financial assistance. Cancer Care's toll-free counseling line provides assistance to cancer patients nationwide. Call (800) 813-HOPE.

The National Alliance of Breast Cancer Organizations (NABCO) is the leading central information resource on breast cancer and a network of 375 breast cancer organizations. The quarterly NABCO News updates professionals and the public about developments in research, programs and policy, and the annual Breast Cancer Resource List compiles books, brochures, hot lines, and video resources useful to patients and professionals, as well as a list of more than 350 local breast cancer support groups nationwide. For more information, contact NABCO at 9 East 37th Street, 10th Floor, New York, NY 10016, (800) 719-9154.

The National Breast Cancer Coalition (NBCC), an advocacy organization, is the national voice seeking public policy change. The NBCC has had a major impact on research funding for breast cancer and on the practice of involving breast cancer survivors in decision making that affects their lives. The NBCC promotes increased breast cancer research, funding, legislation and regulation that benefits breast cancer patients, survivors and women at risk. For more information, contact the NBCC at 1707 L Street NW, Suite 1060, Washington, DC 20036, (202) 296-7477.

pregnant—tamoxifen is not recommended for pregnant or lactating women.

Monitoring Women on Tamoxifen

A discussion about endometrial cancer risk provides a natural transition to a discussion of the optimal medical monitoring of women on tamoxifen. Outside the context of a clinical trial, women taking tamoxifen are, by definition, cancer survivors. As such, they should be reminded of the importance of a low-fat, high-fiber balanced diet, maintaining lean body mass, and the avoidance of exposure to possible disease promoters or carcinogens, first and foremost of which is cigarette smoking.

Presumably, a program to monitor the patient's breast cancer which would usually include routine clinical examinations and mammography is in place, as well as other disease assessment procedures such as bone scans or tumor

Table 1 *(Continued)*

The National Cancer Institute's Cancer Information Service provides information and direction on all aspects of cancer through its regional network. Informational brochures are available without charge. Callers are referred to medical centers and clinical trial programs. Spanish speaking staff members are available. Call (800) 4-CANCER.

The National Coalition for Cancer Survivorship is a national network of independent groups and individuals concerned with survivorship and sources of support for cancer patients and their families. NCCS is a clearinghouse for information and advocates for cancer survivors. 1010 Wayne Ave., 5th Floor, Silver Spring, MD 20910, (301) 650-8868.

The Susan G. Komen Foundation is a national volunteer organization seeking to eradicate breast cancer as a life-threatening disease, working through local chapters and Race for the Cure events in 60 cities. The Foundation is the largest private funder of breast cancer research in the U.S. The Komen Alliance is a comprehensive program for the research, education, diagnosis and treatment of breast disease. Information on screening, BSE, treatment and support is available by calling (800) IM-AWARE or contacting The Susan G. Komen Foundation, Occidental Tower, 5005 LBJ Freeway, Suite 370 LB74, Dallas, TX 75244, (214) 450-1777.

Y-ME National Breast Cancer Organization provides breast cancer information, support and referrals through their national toll-free hot line, (800) 221-2141 (9:00 am to 5:00 pm CST, Monday through Friday, or 24 hours at (312) 986-8228). Trained volunteers, all of whom have had breast cancer, are matched by background and experience to callers whenever possible. Y-ME offers information on establishing local support programs, and has 18 chapters nationwide, in addition to their national headquarters in Chicago. Y-ME has also started a hot line for men whose partners have had breast cancer. Call or write to Y-ME at 212 W. Van Buren Street, Chicago, IL 60607, (312) 986-8228.

marker assays. In addition to reinforcing compliance with this plan, the medical team should outline the following as part of the medical follow-up regimen for patients on tamoxifen:

- All women on tamoxifen should obtain regular gynecological examinations, at least annually
- Patients should specifically indicate to their gynecologists that they are taking tamoxifen. Although this seems an obvious point, we often hear about women, who, unaware of the current recommendation that breast cancer survivors not receive estrogen replacement therapy, avail themselves of topical estrogen preparations without consulting their oncology team.
- Unusual gynecological symptoms, such as bleeding, should be reported to the oncology team and should be immediately investigated by the gynecologist

• A baseline ophthalmologic examination prior to beginning tamoxifen therapy. While this is a useful recommendation for any person, especially older patients, it is based on a recently reported association between tamoxifen and ocular symptoms.[1]

Many women wonder, "How will I know that the tamoxifen is working?" and "What will happen after I stop taking it?" The simple response is that it is presumed to be effective in the absence of recurrent or progressive disease, and its current recommended duration is up to 5 years. Many women correctly perceive, however, that in the adjuvant setting, medical science's current limited ability to accurately identify patients at highest risk for recurrent disease means that we are "overtreating" some women. The benefit/risk tradeoff, understandably, can remain less than completely resolved in the minds of some patients. It might be useful to point out that communication about tamoxifen is ongoing and that any medical developments relevant to the patient's case will be promptly relayed to her. The patient, in turn, should be encouraged to bring questions about the drug to her medical team for satisfactory resolution.

Family Questions About Tamoxifen

The woman with breast cancer may raise questions about the potential merits of tamoxifen for her female relatives. First, it should be emphasized that outside of the NCI-sponsored Breast Cancer Prevention Trial (BCPT), tamoxifen is absolutely not indicated for women at high risk for breast cancer and is not approved for that use. However, her family members may want to learn more about the BCPT, which is exploring tamoxifen's ability to prevent breast cancer in high-risk women, and which, at this writing, is still accruing participants. For more information about this trial, women should be referred to the National Cancer Institute's Cancer Information Service at (800) 4-CANCER.

Second, physicians managing women with breast cancer need to be increasingly prepared to discuss the state of the art of investigating genetic susceptibility to breast cancer, a topic generating interest and excitement among both medical professionals and the public. Many women are not aware, for example, that fewer than 10% of breast cancer cases are currently thought to be the result of an inherited susceptibility. Moreover, although testing for BRCA-1 and BRCA-2 mutations is already available to qualified physicians and their eligible patients, such testing raises many complex ethical, medical, psychosocial, and legal questions. Furthermore, patients should be made aware that the clinical implications (and therefore recommendations for action) of either a positive or negative test result—both for breast cancer survivors and women at risk—are currently unclear and are the subject of continuing study.

Finally, an advantage of referring a patient to information resources for written or videotaped materials about tamoxifen and breast cancer is that these can be shared with family members who are at best concerned and at worst fearful and confused about the prognosis of the woman close to them. An open and thorough discussion with information materials at hand can go a long way toward correcting misperceptions, and offers family members valuable background that can serve them well when they join the patient for office visits.

Despite the fact that breast cancer continues to be many women's greatest health fear, an informed, more actively involved "new patient" is now being seen

Facilitating Good Patient Communication

Whether the topic is tamoxifen or something else, following certain basic guidelines will contribute to the likelihood that the patient/medical professional communication will be a useful and positive one. Although many professionals who routinely advocate for their breast cancer patients follow these guidelines naturally, they are worth repeating:

• Conduct explanatory conversations in person, when the woman is dressed and in an office, rather than in an examining room setting

• Encourage the patient to take notes, bring in a family member or friend, or to tape record these conversations

• Listen carefully to the patient's questions, as well as to other issues that might be implied or revealed

• Answer straightforwardly, balancing reality and hope, and use humor when welcome and appropriate

• If time is limited, the situation should be explained at the outset and the woman should be offered another time to continue the conversation, either in person or on the telephone, or to continue the discussion with another physician, nurse or appropriate member of the medical team.

Caring professionals and breast cancer advocates have made tremendous progress in increasing public awareness of the facts about breast cancer and the need for women to take charge of their health. Continuing media coverage of breast cancer advocacy and scientific developments has contributed to the new approach to breast cancer being taken by an increasing number of women. Despite the fact that breast cancer continues to be many women's greatest health fear, an informed, more actively involved "new patient" is now being seen.

This new breast cancer patient is prepared with background information about the disease and has opinions; requires treatment options; wants good communication and information, and wants the truth; is not passive, and may even hire and fire members of her medical team until she has it configured to her liking; knows the national public policy picture and often belongs to advocacy and information organizations; and expects medical professionals to be advocates for their patients and work for the cause. For medical professionals, communicating well with an involved, informed patient has many satisfactions, which include an improved quality of life and ultimately, the potential for the patient's extended survival.

References

1. Nayfield SG, Gorin MB: Tamoxifen-associated eye disease: A review. *J Clin Oncol* 14:1018-1026, 1996.

Chapter 13

Breast Cancer: Progress Towards the Prospects of Prevention

V. Craig Jordan, PhD, DSc
Director, Breast Cancer Research Program
Robert H. Lurie Cancer Center
Northwestern University Medical School

The Biological Basis for Prevention

The successful use of tamoxifen for the treatment of breast cancer, and the low incidence of side effects observed with the then more than 4.5 million women years of clinical experience (now 8 million), acted as a catalyst to support the use of tamoxifen in normal women at risk for developing breast cancer. During the past two decades, a growing literature on the prevention of rodent mammary cancer supported the clinical use of tamoxifen to prevent breast cancer. As long ago as 1936, Lacassagne[1] predicted that a therapeutic intervention could be developed that would "prevent or antagonize the congestion of oestrone in the breast." Unfortunately, no therapeutic agent was available and all his predictions were based upon the known effect of early oophorectomy on the development of mammary cancer in high incidence strains of mice. Clearly the indiscriminate oophorectomy of young women would be an inappropriate intervention!

Animal studies with tamoxifen were undertaken for two reasons: first, to establish the efficacy of tamoxifen in well described models of carcinogenesis, and secondly, to discover whether tamoxifen would always be an inhibitor, or whether the drug would ever exacerbate tumorigenesis. Two animal model systems have been used extensively: the carcinogen-induced rat mammary carcinoma model and mouse mammary tumor virus (MMTV) infected strains of mice.

The mammary carcinogens dimethylbenzanthracene (DMBA)[2] and N-nitrosomethylurea (NMU)[3] induce tumors in young female rats. The timing of the carcinogenic insult is very important because as the animals age, they become resistant to the mammary carcinogens. Tumorigenesis does not occur in oophorectomized animals and the sooner oophorectomy is performed after the carcinogenic insult, the more effective it is in preventing the development of tumors.[4]

The administration of tamoxifen to carcinogen-treated rats prevents the initiation of carcinogenesis—animals remain tumor-free.[5,6] The short-term administration of tamoxifen at different times after the carcinogenic insult is effective in reducing the number of tumors. Nevertheless, most animals develop at least one tumor after therapy is stopped. In contrast, continuous tamoxifen therapy that is started at 1 month after the administration of carcinogens almost completely inhibits the appearance of mammary tumors (Chapter 3, Figure 7). Under these circumstances, tamoxifen prevents pro-motion and suppresses the appearance of occult disease. In fact, if treatment is stopped prematurely (ie, a 3- to 4-month duration of therapy), the microfoci of transformed cells grow into palpable tumors. Since the timing of initiation in human breast cancer is unknown, and, unlike the laboratory model, not all women will develop tumors, tamoxifen is given to target populations in approved clinical trials to suppress and, hopefully, reverse the promotional effects of estrogen during carcinogenesis.

Until recently, there was a paucity of information about the efficacy of tamoxifen to inhibit mouse mammary tumorigenesis. This was due, in part, to the observation that tamoxifen is estrogenic in short-term tests in oophorectomized and immature mice. However, the finding that long-term tamoxifen therapy renders the oophorectomized mouse vagina and athymic mouse uterus refractory to estrogenic stimuli prompted a reconsideration of the value of tamoxifen as a preventive in mouse mammary tumor models.

High incidence strains of mice that develop mammary tumors are infected with mouse mammary tumor virus (MMTV) (Appendix 1), which is trans-ferred to offspring in the mothers' milk. Tumorigenesis appears to be ovarian dependent, as the highest incidence of tumors appears in females and tumorigenesis can be delayed or prevented, depending on the animal's age at oophorectomy. Steroid hormones activate the proviral MMTV, which, in turn, can initiate an increase in growth factors from the viral integration site Int. 2 in the mouse mammary DNA. Promotion of the initiated cells with steroid hormones and prolactin then completes tumorigenesis. It is clear in the mouse model, *unlike the human*, that early pregnancy promotes the early appearance of mammary tumors.

Long-term tamoxifen therapy, after an early pregnancy to promote tumorigenesis, is equivalent to oophorectomy performed at 4 months, in reducing tumorigenesis by 50% at 14 months of age. Tamoxifen is actually superior to oophorectomy because oophorectomized animals continue to develop tumors, whereas animals previously treated with tamoxifen do not develop any more tumors,[7] even after therapy is stopped.

These initial observations were followed up with another study of tumorigenesis in virgin mice. According to this study design, mice develop mammary tumors during their second year of life. Again, long-term tamoxifen therapy started at 3 months of age is superior to oophorectomy at 3 months. Fifty percent of the oophorectomized animals develop tumors by the third year of life, whereas 90% of tamoxifen-treated mice remain tumor-free.[8] The general conclusions of this study are illustrated in Figure 1.

Overall, results of the mouse model studies are particularly interesting because they have changed our view of the interspecies pharmacology of tamoxifen. Within a few weeks, however, the pharmacology of tamoxifen changes from an estrogen and tamoxifen becomes an antiestrogen. Clearly, an understanding of this process may have important implications for the long-term use of tamoxifen as an adjutant therapy and a preventive.

In mice, long-term tamoxifen therapy started at 3 months of age is superior to oophorectomy at 3 months

Prevention: From the Laboratory to Clinical Trial

Twenty years ago, tamoxifen was shown to prevent the induction[5,6] and promotion[9] of carcinogen-induced mammary cancer in rats. Similarly, tamoxifen prevents the development of mammary cancer induced by ionizing radiation in rats.[10] These laboratory observations, coupled with the emerging preliminary clinical observation that adjuvant tamoxifen would prevent contralateral breast cancer in women,[11] provided a rationale for Dr. Trevor Powles at the Royal Marsden Hospital in England to establish a Vangard study to test whether tamoxifen could prevent breast cancer in high risk women.[12] This chapter will explore the progress that has been achieved in the last decade to answer the question "Does tamoxifen have worth in the prevention of breast cancer in select high-risk women?" This question can only be answered by carefully organized double- blind placebo controlled clinical trials. The design and preliminary results of the three international trials that are currently being conducted—the Royal Marsden Study, the NSABP/NCI study, and and an Italian study—will be described.

Royal Marsden Study

Powles and coworkers have completed recruitment to a pilot randomized placebo controlled trial using tamoxifen 20 mg daily for up to 8 years in healthy women at increased risk of developing breast cancer. The trial was

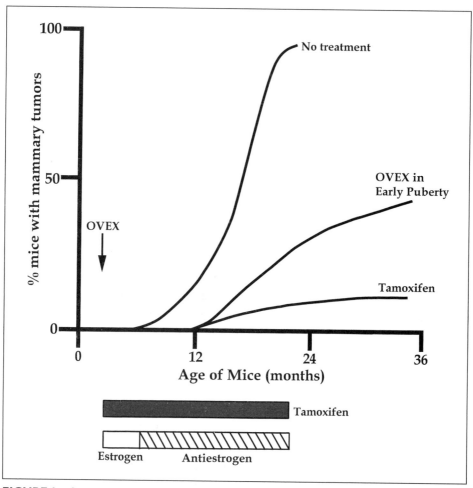

FIGURE I   **Ovariectomy vs tamoxifen in the mouse model**   We compared the effectiveness of ovariectomy (ovex) with long-term tamoxifen treatment in preventing mouse mammary cancer. Virgin mice from inbred high-incidence strains are infected with MMTV and develop mammary tumors spontaneously in the second year of life. The effect of early ovariectomy is to reduce the number of mice that develop tumors. Long-term tamoxifen treatment, however, is even more effective. The black band in the figure describes the effect of tamoxifen in the mouse uterus. The drug is initially able to stimulate an increase in uterine weight (an estrogen-like effect), but with continuous therapy, uterine weight decreases and tamoxifen acts as an antiestrogen.

undertaken to evaluate the problems of accrual, acute symptomatic toxicity, compliance, and safety as a basis for subsequent large national multicenter trials designed to test whether tamoxifen can prevent breast cancer.

From October 1986 until June 1993, 2,012 healthy women with an increased risk of developing breast cancer were recruited.[13] Healthy women aged 30 to 70 years were eligible provided they had a family history of breast cancer on their maternal side with at least one first-degree relative (sister, mother, daughter) who had developed breast cancer before the age of 45, or had developed bilateral breast cancer, or with a first-degree relative, as well as at least one other maternal relative. Women with two affected first-degree relatives of any age were also eligible, as were women with a first-degree relative and a personal history of biopsy for benign breast disease. Women with a history of venous thrombosis, any previous malignancy, or an estimated life expectancy of fewer than 10 years were excluded.

The Marsden group has made an extensive study of gynecological complications associated with tamoxifen treatment in healthy women

Acute symptomatic toxicity was low for participants on tamoxifen or placebo, and compliance remained correspondingly high: 77% of women on tamoxifen and 82% of women on placebo remained on medication at 5 years, as predicted. There was a significant increase in hot flashes (34% vs 20%)–mostly in premenopausal women ($P < 0.005$)—vaginal discharge (16% vs 4%; $P < 0.005$), and menstrual irregularities (14% vs 9%; $P < 0.005$), respectively. Until their report in 1994,[13] the Marsden group observed no thromboembolic episodes; a detailed analysis of other coagulation parameters in a sequential subset of women also found no significant changes in Protein S, Protein C, or cross-linked fibrinogen degradation products. A significant fall in total plasma cholesterol occurs within 3 months and is sustained over 5 years of treatment.[14-16] The decrease affects low density lipoprotein, with no change in apolipoproteins A and B or in high density lipoprotein cholesterol. In contrast, tamoxifen exerts antiestrogenic effects and effects on bone density, depending on menopausal status. In premenopausal women, early findings demonstrate a small but significant ($P < 0.05$) loss of bone in both the lumbar spine and hip at 3 years.[16] It will be most important to evaluate the results at 5 and 8 years of therapy, as current indications suggest bone stabilization rather then continued loss. In contrast, postmenopausal women have increased bone mineral density in the spine ($P < 0.005$) and hip ($P < 0.001$) compared to nontreated women.

Finally, the Marsden group has made an extensive study of gynecological complications associated with tamoxifen treatment in healthy women. Since ovarian and uterine assessment by transvaginal ultrasound became available some time after the start of the trial, many subjects did not have a baseline evaluation. Ovarian screening demonstrated a significantly increased risk ($P < 0.005$) of detecting benign ovarian cysts in premenopausal women who had received tamoxifen for more than 3 months compared to controls. There were no changes in ovarian appearance in postmenopausal women.[13]

A careful examination of the uterus with transvaginal ultrasonography using color Doppler imaging in women taking tamoxifen showed that the organ was usually larger; moreover, women with histological abnormalities had significantly thicker endometria.[17] Of particular interest in this regard is the recent observation that tamoxifen, 20 mg daily, exerts a time-dependent proliferation of endometrial in premenopausal and early postmenopausal women. This effect appears to be mediated by the stromal component, since no cases of cancer or even of epithelial hyperplasia were observed among the tamoxifen-treated group in a recent Italian study with 33 women.[18]

Although the Vangard study is providing invaluable information about the biological effects of tamoxifen in healthy women, the trial was not designed to answer the question of whether tamoxifen will prevent breast cancer. Larger national trials will provide this information. In the United Kingdom, an expanded study has started to enroll 20,000 women nationwide.

NSABP/NCI Study

This study opened in the U.S. and Canada in May 1992, with an accrual goal of 16,000 women to be recruited at 100 North American sites. The study design is illustrated in Figure 2. Those eligible for entry include any woman over the age of 60, or women between the ages of 35 and 59 whose 5-year risk of developing breast cancer, as predicted by the Gail model,[19] equals that of a 60-year old woman. Additionally, any woman over age 35 with a diagnosis of lobular carcinoma in situ (LCIS) treated by biopsy alone is eligible for entry to the study. In the absence of LCIS, the risk factors necessary to enter the study vary with age, such that a 35-year-old woman must have a relative risk (RR), of 5.07, whereas at 45, the RR must be 1.79. Although recruitment to the study has been slow, more than 10,000 women have already been processed and randomized to the study. Health care evaluations are extremely rigorous and, most importantly, all women will have routine endometrial biopsies to evaluate the role of tamoxifen in the detection of pre-existing endometrial conditions.

The breast cancer risk of women already enrolled in the study is extremely high, with no age group below a RR of 4—including the over 60s group. Recruitment is also balanced, with about one third younger than 50 years old, one third between 50 and 60 years old, and one third older than 60 years of age. A full evaluation of lipid and cholesterol profiles is being made, as well as bone density determinations in selected groups. Most importantly, the study will provide the first information about the role of genetic markers in the etiology of breast cancer and will determine whether tamoxifen can have a

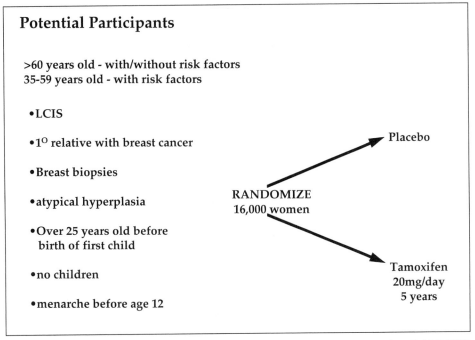

Potential Participants

>60 years old - with/without risk factors
35-59 years old - with risk factors

•LCIS

•1º relative with breast cancer

•Breast biopsies

•atypical hyperplasia

•Over 25 years old before
  birth of first child

•no children

•menarche before age 12

RANDOMIZE
16,000 women

Placebo

Tamoxifen
20mg/day
5 years

FIGURE 2   Study design of the NSABP/NCI chemoprevention trial   The NSABP/NCI chemoprevention trial is underway to test the worth of tamoxifen to reduce the risk of breast cancer in high-risk women. The risk factors for the study population after recruiting 11,000 women is so high that a goal of only 13,000 women needs to be met. This will be accomplished by Summer, 1997.

role to play in the treatment of women who are found to carry somatic mutations in the BRCA-1 gene. Results from this study should be available by the turn of the century.

Italian Study

This study is recruiting 20,000 normal women over the age of 45 to be randomized to 20 mg tamoxifen daily or a placebo for 5 years. Only hysterectomized women are admitted to the trial to avoid issues of pregnancy and endometrial pathologies. To date, more than 4,000 women have been randomized in Italy, and the trial is being opened to other European nations.

Toxicological Concerns

Tamoxifen has been shown, at high doses given for prolonged periods, to produce liver tumors in rats. Such tumors have not been noted in other species and there is no evidence that tamoxifen can cause liver tumors in women. Although millions of women have been exposed to tamoxifen treatment for long periods, only a few (approximately three) liver tumors have been noted worldwide. Since hepatocellular carcinoma is a rare tumor in the Western world (5 per 100,000) any new potentially causative agent like tamoxifen would be quickly implicated in an increase in national statistics. This has not occurred; nevertheless, the issue of the relevance of rat studies for the risk of human liver carcinogenesis has been extensively reviewed.[20,21] It is now clear that tamoxifen effects in rat liver are unique to the rat. It is also clear that if today's concerns about tamoxifen and carcinogenesis had been expressed 20 years ago, tens of thousands of women would have died prematurely from breast cancer because tamoxifen specifically, and antiestrogens in general, would never have been developed.[20] Fortunately, this is not the case, and the successful re-evaluation of tamoxifen safety should reassure both breast cancer patients and healthy participants in new clinical prevention trials.

The World Health Organization, which lists tamoxifen as an *essential* medicine for the treatment of breast cancer, has recently evaluated the evidence for the carcinogenic potential of tamoxifen. As Dr. Assikis pointed out in chapter 9, they concluded that there is insufficient evidence to identify carcinogenic risks other than an elevation in the risk of detecting endometrial cancer. They also stated, however, that no woman should be denied tamoxifen treatment based on this risk because the clinical benefits with respect to treatment of breast cancer far outweigh any toxicological risks.

It must be emphasized, however, that tamoxifen *is not* approved for general use in women without a diagnosis of breast cancer outside approved clinical trials. It is hoped that these clinical trials will provide answers about the risks and benefits, as well as the appropriate role, of tamoxifen as a preventive in women at risk for breast cancer.

A New Approach to Prevention

By the late 1980s, the information we had acquired about the potential beneficial effects of tamoxifen on bones and coronary heart disease could have heralded a new era for the prevention of pathologies associated with the menopause.[22] Hormone replacement therapy can dramatically reduce the risk of coronary heart disease and the development of osteoporosis, but the risks of developing breast cancer are unaltered, or, in some studies, very slightly higher.

We have proposed the development of the ideal antiestrogen that would be targeted to produce specific actions at different sites in a woman's body. The properties of the ideal agent are summarized in Figure 3. Such an agent

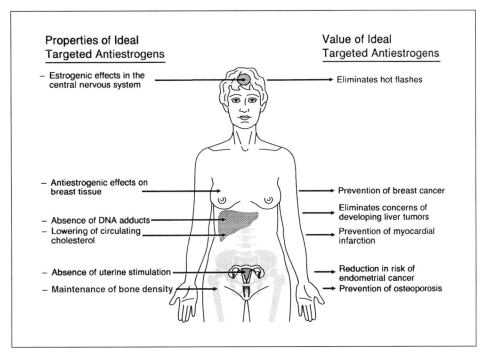

FIGURE 3 **Ideal targeted antiestrogen for postmenopausal women** The ideal agent for hormone replacement therapy should exert estrogenic effects in the brain, to decrease hot flashes and postmenopausal CNS symptoms, to lower cholesterol and reduce coronary heart disease, and to reduce the risk of osteoporosis. It should also, however, act as an antiestrogen in the breast and endometrium to reduce the risk of cancer in both organs.

would have all the benefits of estrogen for the postmenopausal woman but with the added advantage of preventing breast and endometrial cancers.[23]

At present, the two compounds that might fit our criteria, raloxifene and Droloxifene, are being tested clinically for the prevention of osteoporosis in elderly women. It is clear that future drug development in this area will result in appropriate new hormone replacement therapies that might also protect women from breast cancer. A single maintenance medicine for postmenopausal women to prevent osteoporosis and coronary heart disease might conceivably prevent breast and endometrial cancer as a beneficial side effect. There is no doubt that the development of tamoxifen over the past quarter of a century has revolutionized this strategy and the overall prospects for women's health care.

References

1. Lacassagne A: Hormonal pathogenesis of adenocarcinoma of the breast. *Am J Cancer* 14:217-225, 1936.

2. Huggins SC, Grand LC, Brillantes FP: Mammary cancer induced by a single feeding of polynuclear hydrocarbons and their suppression. *Nature* 189:204-207, 1962.

3. Gullino PM, Pettigrew HN, Grantham FH: N-Nitrosomethyurea as mammary gland carcinogen in rats. *J Natl Cancer Inst* 54:401-414, 1975.

4. Dao TL: The role of ovarian hormones in initiating the induction of mammary cancer in rats by polynuclear hydrocarbons. *Cancer Res* 22:973-981, 1962.

5. Jordan VC: Antitumour activity of the antioestrogen ICI 46,474 (tamoxifen) in the dimethylbenzanthracene (DMBA) induced rat mammary carcinoma model. *J Steroid Biochem* 5:354, 1974.

6. Jordan VC: Effect of tamoxifen (ICI 46,474) on initiation and growth of DMBA-induced rat mammary carcinomata. *Eur J Cancer* 12:419-425, 1976.

7. Jordan VC, Lababidi MK, Mirecki DM: The antiestrogenic and antitumor properties of prolonged tamoxifen therapy in C3H/OUJ mice. *Eur J Cancer* 26:718-721, 1990.

8. Jordan VC, Lababidi MK, Langan Fahey S: Suppression of mouse mammary tumorigenesis by long term tamoxifen therapy. *J Natl Cancer Inst* 83:492-496, 1991.

9. Jordan VC, Allen KE, Dix CJ: Pharmacology of tamoxifen in laboratory animals. *Cancer Treat Rep* 64:745-759, 1980.

10. Welsch CW, Goodrich-Smith M, Brown CK, et al: Effect of an estrogen antagonist (tamoxifen) on the initiation and progression of gamma radiation-induced mammary tumors in female Sprague-Dawley rats. *Eur J Cancer* 17:1255-1258, 1981.

11. Cuzick J, Baum M: Tamoxifen and contralateral breast cancer. *Lancet* 2:282, 1985.

12. Powles TJ, Hardy JR, Ashley SE, et al: A pilot trial to evaluate the acute toxicity and feasibility of tamoxifen for prevention of breast cancer. *Br J Cancer* 60:126-133, 1989.

13. Powles TJ, Jones AL, Ashley SE, et al: The Royal Marsden Hospital pilot tamoxifen chemoprevention trial. *Breast Cancer Res Treat* 31:73-82, 1994.

14. Jones AL, Powles TJ, Treleaven J, et al: Haemostatic changes and thromboembolic risk during tamoxifen therapy in normal women. *Br J Cancer* 66:744-747, 1992.

15. Powles TJ, Tillyer CP, Jones AL, et al: Prevention of breast cancer with tamoxifen: An update on the Royal Marsden pilot program. *Eur J Cancer* 26:680-684, 1990.

16. Powles TJ, Hickish T, Kanis JA, et al: Effect of tamoxifen on bone mineral density measured by dual-energy X ray absorptiometry in healthy premenopausal and post-menopausal women. *J Clin Oncol* 14:78-84, 1996.

17. Kedar RP, Bourne TH, Powles TJ, et al: Effects of tamoxifen on uterus and ovaries of postmenopausal women in a randomized breast cancer prevention trial. *Lancet* 343:1318-1321, 1994.

18. Decensi A, Fontant V, Bruno S et al 1996. Effect of tamoxifen on endometrial proliferation. *J Clin Oncol* 14:434-440.

19. Gail MH, Brinton LA, Byar DP, et al: Projecting individualized probabilities of

developing breast cancer for white females who are being examined annually. *J Natl Cancer Inst* 81:1879-1886, 1989.

20. Jordan VC: What if tamoxifen (ICI 46,474) had been found to produce liver tumors in rats in 1973? *Ann Oncol* 6:29-34, 1995.

21. Jordan VC: Tamoxifen and tumorigenicity: A predictable concern. *J Natl Cancer Inst* 87:623-626, 1995.

22. Lerner LJ, Jordan VC: Development of antiestrogens and their use in breast cancer: Eighth Cain Memorial Award Lecture. *Cancer Res* 50:4177-4189, 1990.

23. Tonetti DA, Jordan VC: Targeted antiestrogens to treat and prevent diseases in women. *Mol Med Today* 2:218-223, 1996.

This section of the book is dedicated to Amy Langer
in tribute to her great courage

Chapter 14

A Roundtable Discussion: Questions and Answers About Tamoxifen

Jack Gentile, President, PRR, Inc.: "In addition to the journal *ONCOLOGY*, our company publishes two news magazines, *Oncology News International* for cancer specialists and *Primary Care & Cancer* for primary care physicians. The latter two publications both offer their audiences an opportunity to write in and ask our panel of experts any questions they have relating to cancer.

"The most common questions we have received over the past couple of years from both our cancer specialty audience and the primary care physicians relate to the use of tamoxifen (Nolvadex) in breast cancer patients. The vast amount of reporting on tamoxifen in both professional publications and the popular media has inevitably led to confusion and misinformation regarding the use of this drug. It is our hope that this roundtable discussion, which brings together seven breast cancer experts and a representative from a national breast cancer patient group, will offer a clearer picture of the role of tamoxifen in breast cancer and its proper use. Dr. V. Craig Jordan of Northwestern University will moderate the discussion."

◀ **Participants in the 1995 San Antonio Roundtable** on Tamoxifen sponsored by PRR, Inc., publishers of the journal ONCOLOGY, Oncology News International, Primary Care & Cancer, and Cancer Management. From left to right, top (1): Amy Langer (large photo), Executive Director of the National Association of Breast Cancer Organizations; (2) Monica Morrow, MD, of Northwestern University Medical School; (3) C. Kent Osborne, MD, of the University of Texas Health Science Center, San Antonio; (4) Norman Wolmark, MD, of the National Surgical Adjuvant Breast and Bowel Project (NSABP); (5) I. Craig Henderson, MD, of the University of California, San Francisco; (6) the editor of this book, V. Craig Jordan, PhD, DSc, of Northwestern University Medical School; (7) Richard Barakat, MD, of Memorial Sloan-Kettering Cancer Center; (8) a view of the dais. Shown are (l to r) C. Kent Osborne, Richard Barakat, V. Craig Jordan, Monica Morrow, Amy Langer, and Joseph Ragaz. Not shown are Norman Wolmark and I. Craig Henderson. (9) Joseph Ragaz, MD, of the British Columbia Cancer Agency.

Dr. V. Craig Jordan: "Over the past 25 years, we have seen dramatic developments in the use of tamoxifen, and I think it is fair to say that it is the endocrine therapy of choice for selected patients with all stages of breast cancer. There has been a clear-cut demonstration of its biological efficacy in the clinic, and obviously some troublesome side effects and concerns as well. The goal of this roundtable discussion is to put these side effects into perspective and to weigh the pros and cons of tamoxifen use from the patient's point of view. I have prepared a number of questions to ask the panel and will also take questions from the audience.

1. What are the major concerns about tamoxifen voiced by breast cancer patients, and how do you balance the possible side effects against the known benefits?

Dr. Jordan: "The first question involves the concerns about tamoxifen that physicians hear from their patients and that cancer survivors express within their patient organizations. Dr. Morrow, what has been your experience in this regard?"

Dr. Monica Morrow: "Five years ago, most patients' concerns were what I would consider the primary and appropriate concerns, namely, what will tamoxifen do to keep me from dying of breast cancer? More recently, secondary to adverse publicity surrounding the Breast Cancer Prevention Trial (BCPT) [in this trial, women at high risk for breast cancer are being randomized to receive tamoxifen or placebo for 5 years] and the National Surgical Adjuvant Breast and Bowel Project (NSABP) studies, the main issue now among patients is side effects, primarily endometrial cancer, but also, to a much lesser extent, liver cancer and, among premenopausal women, the misconception that tamoxifen will induce premature menopause.

"I put these concerns into perspective by stressing the risk-to-benefit ratio of tamoxifen use. The beneficial effects on survival of breast cancer patients who take tamoxifen far outweigh the possible adverse effects."

Ms. Amy S. Langer: "As knowledge of a drug's benefits increases over the years, so does knowledge of its side effects, and this is often what the media pick up. I think that some of the concerns about endometrial cancer raised by the media have been quite distorted. In fact, there have been very few cases of endometrial cancer reported in clinical trials of tamoxifen. It is incumbent on all of us to be sure that the facts about tamoxifen, including updated information from trials and the Oxford meta-analysis, are widely disseminated, and that we try to convince the media of their crucial role in letting patients know the proven beneficial effects of tamoxifen use.

Table I

Roundtable Participants

Moderator: **V. Craig Jordan, PhD, DSc**   Director, Breast Cancer Research Program, Robert H. Lurie Cancer Center, Northwestern University Medical School

Richard R. Barakat, MD   Assistant Attending Surgeon, Gynecology Service, Memorial Sloan-Kettering Cancer Center

I. Craig Henderson, MD   Adjunct Professor of Medicine, University of California, San Francisco

Amy S. Langer   Executive Director, National Alliance of Breast Cancer Organizations (NABCO)

Monica Morrow, MD   Director, Lynn Sage Comprehensive Breast Program, Northwestern University Medical School

C. Kent Osborne, MD   AB Alexander Distinguished Chair and Chief of Medical Oncology, University of Texas Health Science Center, San Antonio

Joseph Ragaz, MD   Senior Medical Oncologist, Vancouver Cancer Centre, British Columbia Cancer Agency, University of British Columbia

Norman Wolmark, MD   Chairman, Department of Human Oncology, Medical College of Pennsylvania/Hahnemann University, Allegheny Campus, Pittsburgh, and Chairman of the National Surgical Adjuvant Breast and Bowel Project (NSABP)

"When women taking tamoxifen call the National Association of Breast Cancer Organizations (NABCO) with concerns about endometrial cancer, we stress the importance of routine gynecologic surveillance. We also prefer to emphasize the positive data from the NSABP B-14 trial—that tamoxifen in node-negative breast cancer is clearly beneficial, compared with no tamoxifen, and that 5 years' duration is now the standard."

Dr. C. Kent Osborne: "I think that patient concerns about tamoxifen side effects stem largely from misinformation that they have heard, not only from the media but also from physicians who may not understand the dual effects of antiestrogens like tamoxifen. These drugs have beneficial estrogen-agonist properties in some tissues and antagonist properties in the breast. Lacking this understanding, some patients and physicians may fear, incorrectly, that tamoxifen will have undesirable antiestrogen effects on cholesterol or bone density, or they may overestimate the risk of endometrial cancer. The net result of these misunderstandings is that women may stop taking the drug prematurely, in some cases without telling their physician."

2. What do the clinical trials, specifically NSABP B-14, show about the question of endometrial cancer?

Dr. Jordan: I would like to specifically address the issue of increased risk of endometrial cancer risk because it seems to be the dominant negative side effect of tamoxifen. Dr. Wolmark, can you discuss the NSABP findings?"

Dr. Norman Wolmark: "The question of endometrial cancers should not be trivialized, and patients who take tamoxifen need to be apprised of the risk, but I also think that the risk needs to be placed in perspective. Tamoxifen is an extremely effective, relatively nontoxic drug in the treatment of breast cancer, particularly in the adjuvant setting. The NSABP protocol B-14, a randomized prospective trial, attempted to determine the benefit of tamoxifen in a specific subset of women: those with histologically negative nodes whose tumors were estrogen receptor (ER)-positive.

"Ten-year results now indicate that there is an unequivocal and significant prolongation of disease-free survival with tamoxifen (68%) vs placebo (57%). Overall survival was also increased with tamoxifen use: from 75% for placebo to 78% for tamoxifen, a statistically significant increase. So basically we have a prolongation in survival and a reduction in recurrence rate. This has to be weighed against the negative aspects, and the primary negative aspect is the occurrence of endometrial cancer.

"In the entire trial (1,400 women in each arm), there were 21 cases of endometrial cancer in patients randomized to receive tamoxifen. Certainly, that is more than would occur in the general, untreated, age-matched population, but to put it into perspective, it is certainly no more than would occur in women who are over age 50 and receiving unopposed estrogen replacement therapy.

"Overall, the benefits of tamoxifen in this population far outweigh the risks. And I think that basically women at large have been done a disservice by media reports of the risks of tamoxifen taken out of context of the benefits."

Dr. Jordan: "I would like to ask Dr. Ragaz how the endometrial cancer controversy is viewed in Canada?"

Dr. Joseph Ragaz: "Using data from the Canadian Registry, we estimated the late effects of tamoxifen on overall mortality. Calculations were done for each age cohort taking four principal conditions associated with tamoxifen effect: contralateral breast cancer, cardiac events, uterine cancer, and thromboembolic phenomena. Results have shown that, despite moderate excess of mortality from uterine cancer and thromboembolic events, there was a more substantial mortality reduction from contralateral breast cancer and cardiac events. The main conclusion of our work indicates that despite a dramatic rise in uterine cancer risk, mortality is affected marginally, as only small absolute numbers will be affected. On the other hand, while only moderate RR reductions are seen for contralateral breast cancer and cardiac events, mortality will be reduced more significantly as large numbers across whole populations are affected.

The risk of endometrial cancer has to be emphasized, but it should not overshadow the potential benefit of tamoxifen in reducing overall mortality

"On the other hand, while the increase in uterine cancer mortality is large, the absolute number of women affected is very small. In absolute terms, for each uterine cancer induced by tamoxifen, there would be a 5% to 10% reduction in breast cancer and cardiac mortality. So the risk of endometrial cancer is vastly overwhelmed by the benefits of tamoxifen when you look at its potential to improve late mortality.

"These data do not mean we should underestimate the importance of the risk of endometrial cancer. On the contrary, our knowledge of the increased risk should lead to improved screening, which may eventually lead to reductions in endometrial cancer mortality. So the risk of endometrial cancer has to be emphasized, but it should not overshadow the potential benefit of tamoxifen in reducing overall mortality."

3. Is endometrial cancer that occurs during tamoxifen therapy more aggressive?

Dr. Jordan: "I think one of the big issues with the endometrial cancer question really occurred in the early 1990s with the publication of an article based on the Yale-New Haven database suggesting that endometrial cancers in women who had taken tamoxifen were more aggressive. I would like to ask Dr. Barakat about his study of this issue at Memorial Sloan-Kettering Cancer Center, to be followed by some comments from Dr. Wolmark about the grade and stage of the endometrial cancers seen in the B-14 trial."

Dr. Richard R. Barakat: "When endometrial cancer does occur in women on tamoxifen, it is not more aggressive, as was suggested by the review of the Yale-New Haven tumor registry. This report prompted us to review Memorial Sloan-Kettering's registry of breast cancer patients to specifically examine those who subsequently developed cancer of the uterus.

"We identified 27 patients who received tamoxifen and developed endometrial cancer after a breast cancer diagnosis. The results showed that 75% to 80% of the endometrial cancers in the tamoxifen group were low-grade, stage I, highly curable lesions, a distribution similar to that seen in the 50 breast cancer patients from the registry who had developed endometrial cancer but had not taken tamoxifen. This is also what you see in the general population—75% to 80% of endometrial cancers are confined to the uterus, stage I disease, usually with a low grade."

Dr. Wolmark: "Based on the NSABP experience, there is no evidence that the endometrial cancers found in women on tamoxifen are different from those that develop in patients who do not receive tamoxifen, with the majority of such lesions being low grade and confined. That's not to say there won't be deaths resulting from endometrial cancer that develops while taking tamoxifen, but we have not seen anything unique about endometrial cancers that occur in tamoxifen patients, relative to histology, distribution, or level of aggressiveness."

Dr. Jordan: "I recently published, with my colleague at Northwestern, Dr. Vasilios Assikis, a review of international data that backs up both of the previous two speakers. We found, essentially, that the grade and stage of endometrial cancers associated with tamoxifen use are in exactly the same proportions as those seen in SEER data throughout the United States. So I think it is fair to say that all of the evidence that we have available to us now has been contrary to that single report of more aggressive endometrial cancers with tamoxifen use from the Yale-New Haven database."

4. Can anything be done to prevent the development of endometrial cancer during tamoxifen therapy or to diagnose it earlier?

Dr. Jordan: "Before we leave the endometrial cancer controversy, I would like to ask the panel to comment on any measures that can be taken to avoid the development of endometrial cancer in patients taking tamoxifen or to diagnose cases earlier. For example, the literature suggests that administration of a progestin can prevent hot flashes and postmenopausal symptoms. Is it possible, then, that progestins could be used to help prevent endometrial cancer in patients taking tamoxifen? I'll ask our gynecologist, Dr. Barakat, to respond."

Dr. Barakat: "As you know, there is really no proven medical screening for endometrial cancer, and there are many problems with the use of routine endometrial biopsies, ultrasonography, and vaginal sonography. In terms of progestins, we know they can be used to prevent the untoward effects of estrogen replacement therapy on the uterus, but whether we can give them safely with tamoxifen remains to be shown.

"My understanding is that there is not a lot of concern about giving progestins to women with breast cancer, but there are preclinical data showing that it may have an adverse effect in terms of their breast cancer. Whether local progestin administration, for example, intrauterine progestin for a limited time, is beneficial remains to be proved. The biggest problem that I can see with giving women progestins comes from our medical oncology colleagues who really don't want us to use these agents, especially in high doses, in women with a history of breast cancer."

In terms of the overall quality of life of patients, we are probably on the verge of doing more harm than good by sending them for excessive endometrial screening

Dr. Osborne: "We really don't know how to monitor patients on tamoxifen for endometrial cancer and we certainly don't know how to prevent it. However, this is being studied in the cooperative groups, and the Southwest Oncology Group (SWOG) is planning a trial to see whether progestins will reduce the incidence of endometrial cancer and whether screening with vaginal ultrasound, hysteroscopy, and biopsies will help in assessing premalignant changes in the uterus. So hopefully in the next year or so information will become available from these and other trials, and we'll have a better feel for how best to monitor these patients and to catch endometrial cancer early if it does occur.

"What bothers me most right now is that I think we've blown this whole thing out of proportion and by performing endometrial screening, we are substantially increasing the cost of giving adjuvant tamoxifen with no evidence that the extra tests have any benefit. In terms of the overall quality of life of patients, we are probably on the verge of doing more harm than good by sending them for excessive endometrial testing."

Dr. Ragaz: "In British Columbia, our community oncologists do not accept universally that progestin use improves hot flashes and other side effects of tamoxifen. The prevalent opinion is that estrogen is beneficial. However, the issue of uterine cancer is forcing the issue of progestin use. We have proposed a randomized trial in breast cancer survivors of tamoxifen plus estrogen vs tamoxifen plus a progestin, and I know that ECOG is also planning a randomized study of similar design. If this issue is to be addressed properly, it should be done within the context of randomized studies."

Ms. Langer: "As a nonphysician, I would just remind all of us that a very good way to avoid endometrial cancer is not to have an endometrium. In fact, in this country, more than one third of women who are at the age of increased breast cancer risk tend to be hysterectomized. So we should bear in mind that because of the natural patterns of medical care, a substantial proportion of women with breast cancer are not at risk of endometrial cancer because, like women of the same age in the general population, they may have already had a hysterectomy."

Dr. Morrow: "We don't really know what constitutes cost-effective screening for endometrial cancer and, as has been suggested, this needs to be studied. One thing that everyone can agree on, however, is that women who are about to start tamoxifen should have a careful gynecologist examination to exclude preexisting endometrial cancer. In every report of tamoxifen-related endometrial cancer in the literature, there are many cases that occur within 2 to 6 months of starting the drug, and these are clearly not drug-induced cases. This is a group of patients who should be screened out prior to starting therapy."

5. Is there an increased risk of liver cancer from tamoxifen use?

Dr. Jordan: "Scientific observations from several years ago showed development of liver cancers in rats given large doses of tamoxifen. However, if these animal doses are translated into human doses, it would be the equivalent of a 14-year-old female taking 80 tamoxifen tablets daily until age 45 or 50. Dr. Wolmark, has increased liver toxicity been seen in any clinical trials?"

Dr. Wolmark: "Analysis of the cumulative data of the NSABP trials has shown no increased incidence of gastrointestinal cancers, including liver cancers, even with 10 years of tamoxifen use."

Dr. I. Craig Henderson: "The increased risks of liver cancer with tamoxifen use, if any, is so small that I tell my patients it is about what you would expect with the use of birth control pills."

Dr. Ragaz: "A 15-year review of the British Columbia tumor registry involving more than 27,000 breast cancer patients, most of whom had received tamoxifen, found 24 cases of gallbladder common duct cancer and five cases of liver disease, very similar to what we've seen in the population at large."

Ms. Langer: "I think those of us familiar with the data are reassured about liver cancer, but we do know that tamoxifen can induce some liver changes that are not easily interpretable by patients or their community physicians. Could someone comment on that?"

As a physician seeing tamoxifen patients for the past 20 years, I have never seen clinically significant eye changes associated with tamoxifen use

Dr. Osborne: "Liver function abnormalities occasionally show up in the blood tests that some of us obtain every 6 months in following these patients, but in my experience it is uncommon. I inform patients about the potential for some liver damage, but I have not seen a clinically important ramification of these liver abnormalities, and have never had to stop tamoxifen because of it. With almost any drug, there are going to be some patients who cannot tolerate it because of elevated liver function tests, but it is rare."

Dr. Wolmark: "In the NSABP trials, we have not seen a difference in liver dysfunction between patients on tamoxifen and those on placebo."

6. Are there any concerns about tamoxifen's effects on the eyes?

Dr. Jordan: "I was surprised to learn that there are some concerns about possible adverse effects of tamoxifen use on the eyes. The package insert states that tamoxifen has the potential to cause cataracts and retinal problems. What information is there in the literature about eye problems, and do you feel that this is a concern for your patients? Dr. Osborne?"

Dr. Osborne: "This question is being addressed in the Breast Cancer Prevention Trial and although the results have not yet been disclosed, we are not seeing any problems that would warrant alterations of that trial. We have not seen an increased incidence of cataracts. Those changes that have been noted are mainly ophthalmologic curiosities rather than any condition that would impair vision or lead to any kind of permanent dysfunction of the eye. So like other tamoxifen side effects, that too has been played out of proportion.

"Some early NCI trials of tamoxifen back in the early 1970s, in which patients received high doses for a long time period, did generate some eye changes, but only at the very high doses being given and only with prolonged treatment. Since then, there have been a few scattered studies suggesting that minor changes, corneal opacities and so on, may occur. But in carefully done studies with careful ophthalmologic examination, these have not turned out to be significant. And certainly, as a physician seeing tamoxifen patients for the past 20 years, I have never seen clinically significant eye changes associated with tamoxifen use."

Dr. Morrow: "I agree. I think the concern came from uncontrolled, relatively anecdotal reports in older women who had aggressive screening. It was not surprising that some eye problems were found in these patients."

Dr. Henderson: "I think Dr. Osborne summarized it beautifully. The initial findings from the NCI were real, but the doses were very high, about 100 mg BID. I think all the other observations are really anecdotal and a remarkably small number when you consider the number of patient-years of follow-up we have on this drug—about 100 cases in 7 million woman-years of experience."

Dr. Jordan: "Yes, they were really huge doses. And I think it was something like 100 anecdotal cases in about 7 million woman-years of tamoxifen."

Dr. Ragaz: "We submitted about 80 of our long-term tamoxifen patients to regular ophthalmologic examination and found that up to 10% had mild keratopathy and gritty eyes (dry eyes). So our small uncontrolled sample indicates that there may be some temporary, self-limiting keratopathy, but we did not see any lens problems."

7. What are the possible noncancer benefits of tamoxifen that you discuss with your patients, and is there evidence in the literature to support these discussions?

Dr. Jordan: "I would like to turn now to a question about other noncancer beneficial effects of tamoxifen and how they are integrated into the patient discussion. Dr. Morrow, could you comment?"

Dr. Morrow: "The risk-to-benefit ratio for the use of adjuvant tamoxifen therapy should be considered outside of the narrow confines of survival or death from metastatic breast cancer. For women with node-positive breast cancer, the overwhelming force of mortality is always the breast cancer, but in women with smaller, node-negative breast cancers, other causes of mortality—eg, cardiovascular disease, complications of osteoporosis, and other cancers—are a bigger issue.

"Data suggest that besides prevention of breast cancer recurrence, tamoxifen has additional benefits that might impact overall survival. Namely, it can lower cholesterol levels and reduce hospital admissions for cardiovascular disease, as demonstrated in the Stockholm trial, and, as shown in the Scottish studies, even in older women, tamoxifen may reduce mortality from cardiovascular disease.

"On the other hand, perhaps these findings are not absolute. The recent overview analysis of adjuvant tamoxifen from the Early Breast Cancer Trialists' Collaborative Group failed to demonstrate a reduction in non-breast cancer mortality with use of tamoxifen."

Data suggest that besides prevention of breast cancer recurrence, tamoxifen has additional benefits that might impact overall survival

Dr. Henderson: "I was a little disconcerted with the overview analysis results showing no reduction in non-breast cancer mortality with tamoxifen use, and I remain unconvinced that the current analysis provides the final word on the subject. The contributions of various trials to the overview have not been analyzed. For example, this effect on non-breast cancer mortality, which was rather striking at the last overview analysis, may be less so now because of the inclusion of many more trials with shorter follow-up.

"As Dr. Morrow said, I think that for breast cancer patients with a low risk of recurrence, these issues are very important in the decision to take tamoxifen."

Dr. Jordan: "Patients in many of the trials in the meta-analysis have not necessarily used tamoxifen for 5 years, whereas the data on hormone replacement therapy in postmenopausal women suggest that longer is better in regard to maintaining protection against cardiovascular disease."

Dr. Osborne: "I think we should certainly raise these issues with patients and tell them that there may be additional ancillary benefits of tamoxifen use, even though the long-term benefits are uncertain."

Dr. Wolmark: "The current Breast Cancer Prevention Trial (BCPT), along with its primary end point of breast cancer prevention, has other specific end points designed to measure the benefit of tamoxifen relative to osteoporosis (prevention of fractures) and cardiovascular disease (reduction in cardiovascular deaths). This is an extremely important trial; 11,000 women, out of a planned 16,000, [now 12,400 of 13,000] have already been randomized. These are women who do not have breast cancer but are at high risk for developing the disease, either because they are over age 60, they have one or more first-degree blood relatives who have had breast cancer, or they have had lobular carcinoma in situ treated by lumpectomy alone."

8. What are the breast cancer benefits of tamoxifen besides increased survival?

Dr. Jordan: "There are other important cancer-related benefits associated with tamoxifen that we have not yet addressed, and I'll ask Dr. Wolmark to review these."

Dr. Wolmark: "Two other important benefits associated with tamoxifen beyond any survival benefits are the reduction in the incidence of contralateral breast cancer and the prevention of breast cancer recurrence in patients who have had lumpectomies.

"In all of the NSABP studies in which we've used tamoxifen as an adjunct of the treatment of breast cancer, we've noted that the incidence of breast cancer in the opposite breast has been reduced by 40% to 50%. It was this observation that provided the background and justification to start the Breast Cancer Prevention Trial (BCPT).

"Use of tamoxifen in breast conservation patients who have received radiotherapy reduces the risk of recurrence by an additional 3% at 10 years. So the chances of that women keeping that breast is significantly improved when tamoxifen or chemotherapy is added to the regimen. I think this is an important benefit of tamoxifen that is totally overlooked in most studies that assess the risk-to-benefit ratio."

Dr. Morrow: "Whether or not tamoxifen use improves survival in women who have had breast conservation, it adds to the quality of life of these patients, since those who chose breast preservation did so because they wanted to keep their breast."

9. What are the concerns of giving tamoxifen in the premenopausal patient?

Dr. Jordan: "I would like now to ask the panel about the use of tamoxifen in the premenopausal patient. Concerns have been raised about high circulating levels of estradiol that sometimes cause irregular menstrual cycles. What are your thoughts about the risks-to-benefits ratio of tamoxifen in premenopausal patients? Dr. Osborne?"

Dr. Osborne: "I would not be very concerned about the menstrual irregularities. They do occur in maybe 20% or so of patients, but this is not a major problem. A potential problem is that many patients on tamoxifen do get elevated estradiol levels, significantly elevated in some cases, and there is the concern that these high levels may make the tamoxifen less effective by competing with tamoxifen molecules for the estrogen receptors.

"There have been no adequate studies to address this potential problem, in which tumors would be biopsied to measure the amount of estrogen and the amount of tamoxifen in the tumor. These kinds of studies are needed to really pin this down. However, clinical results are coming out suggesting that tamoxifen is still effective in premenopausal women despite this rise in estrogen levels.

"There are four randomized trials in metastatic breast cancer comparing tamoxifen with ovarian ablation. These are all small trials, but when you pool the information, the relative effectiveness of tamoxifen in premenopausal women is in the same ball park as that of ovarian ablation. The recent meta-analysis also suggests that adjuvant tamoxifen in estrogen-receptor-positive premenopausal patients who have not received chemotherapy does offer a disease-free and overall survival advantage. So I think that while there may be some concerns about this rising estrogen level in young women, it doesn't appear to be important as a cause of resistance to the drug."

The important aspect of this issue is not the theoretical objections to using tamoxifen in premenopausal women, but the actual effects of its use in prolonging disease-free and overall survival

Dr. Wolmark: "I think the important aspect of this issue is not the theoretical objections to using tamoxifen in premenopausal women, but the actual effects of its use in prolonging disease-free and overall survival. The NSABP protocol B-14 assessed tamoxifen in both pre- and postmenopausal women with node-negative, receptor-positive disease. The study showed absolutely no difference in the responsiveness to tamoxifen based on age. The premenopausal women had prolongation of disease-free and overall survival just as did the postmenopausal women. So I think that the suggestion that premenopausal patients are tamoxifen-resistant is not borne out by the data from randomized clinical trials.

"I think a lot of the concerns were based on the earlier trials from node-positive patients, from which people concluded that adding tamoxifen to chemotherapy in young premenopausal women was not as effective as adding tamoxifen to chemotherapy in patients over age 50. This still needs to be assessed today, but certainly from the node-negative trials there is no suggestion that there is a relationship between patient age and tamoxifen benefit."

Dr. Jordan: "Dr. Morrow, you mentioned earlier that your younger patients were concerned about the possibility of tamoxifen-induced menopause. Do you want to elaborate on that?"

Dr. Morrow: "Certainly there is a percentage of women taking tamoxifen who will get menstrual irregularity, but I think it is important to remember that for the majority of premenopausal women, tamoxifen actually acts as a stimulant to ovulation. In fact, the agent had a brief life as a fertility drug. So premenopausal women who are on tamoxifen need to be cautioned that pregnancy is a possibility and that barrier contraception should be used."

Dr. Jordan: "Dr. Henderson, would you like to comment on the possibility of tamoxifen resistance in younger women?"

Dr. Henderson: "I think clearly the question of tamoxifen resistance in premenopausal patients with metastatic breast cancer is a moot point. You can tell whether a patient responds, and if she is responding, then therapy should be continued. In the adjuvant setting, however, it is a bit more complicated. I don't think there is any question abut that adjuvant tamoxifen imparts substantial benefits when used in premenopausal women. It would appear from the most recent overview that the use of tamoxifen alone produces a benefit of the same magnitude as seen in postmenopausal women.

"The unanswered questions, however, revolve around two points. One, is tamoxifen really equivalent to chemotherapy in younger women? Indirect comparison suggests that it might be. Two, is it equivalent to oophorectomy? We've done several randomized trials in patients with metastatic breast cancer. None of them is completely reliable, since those physicians who believed ovarian ablation was preferable failed to submit their patients for tamoxifen therapy and vice versa. But the results do suggest a trend in favor of ovarian ablation.

"A third question, which may be of the greatest practical importance, is whether the optimal duration of adjuvant tamoxifen may be different in younger and older women. Indirect comparisons of duration seem to show that for older women there is clearly a difference between 2 years and 1 year of tamoxifen, but it's not so clear that there is a difference between, say, 5 years and 2 or 3 years. Among younger women, however, there clearly is very little or no benefit seen with 1 year of tamoxifen, and it is really only when we began using tamoxifen for 5 years, particularly in the NSABP trials, that we established without question that there was a benefit in the younger women.

"So I think this is a question that remains open. I think that there is probably going to be an optimal duration of treatment with tamoxifen, and I think it may differ for younger and older women."

10. What can be said about the appropriate duration of tamoxifen?

Dr. Jordan: "That is a good point, and it leads into the next discussion: the issue of how long tamoxifen should be given. The National Cancer Institute has recommended that physicians limit tamoxifen use in the treatment of early breast cancer to 5 years in clinical practice. The NCI announcement came on the heels of the decision by the NSABP to stop clinical trial B-14 comparing 5 and 10 years of tamoxifen use after surgery in women with node-negative, ER-positive breast cancer.

We would like to think that because node-positive patients have a slightly worse prognosis that giving more tamoxifen is better, but that may well not be the case

"In this trial, 1,172 women who had been on tamoxifen for 5 years and had not relapsed were randomized a second time to either 5 more years of tamoxifen, 20 mg/day, or placebo. After 4 years of follow-up, 92% of the placebo group were alive and free of disease, compared with 86% of the group scheduled to receive 10 years of tamoxifen.

"The NSABP study is really only the first piece of evidence as to what might be the optimal duration for the pre- and postmenopausal, ER-positive, node-negative woman. And it looks like 5 years may be the right way to go, but the optimal duration might be different in node-positive women. Dr. Osborne, would you comment on this issue?"

Dr. Osborne: "Ideas on tamoxifen duration have changed over the last 10 years. Initially, it was felt that since tamoxifen seemed to be predominantly a cytostatic agent, it might be best to continue the drug for a longer period of time, maybe indefinitely. Now, additional data, both clinical and laboratory, are accumulating to suggest that we may have been wrong in our initial hypothesis. Molecular biology studies suggest that, in some cases, tamoxifen, an antiestrogen, can become a stimulatory agent in the breast. It raises the possibility that there may be an optimal duration for tamoxifen in the adjuvant situation, and it may be shorter than we might have imagined before."

Dr. Jordan: "I would like to emphasize that the NSABP results should be provided as evidence for that particular group of patients only—ER-positive, node-negative women. I would like to see a more definitive comparison in different stages of the disease and in both pre- and postmenopausal women, and such efforts are currently underway. But, unfortunately, there cannot be a definitive answer given at this point in time for all stages of the disease."

Dr. Osborne: "We would like to think that because node-positive patients have a slightly worse prognosis that giving more tamoxifen is better, but that may well not be the case. And I think outside of a clinical research trial, I wouldn't give the agent for more than 5 years, even in node-positive patients.

"The NSABP trial is not alone in showing that extending tamoxifen duration beyond 5 years adds no further benefit. There is a smaller trial from Scotland that showed similar results, and the Scottish trial included both node-negative and node-positive patients."

Dr. Morrow: "The duration question is not completely answered, and we have traditionally been relatively reluctant to stop tamoxifen in node-positive patients who are disease free. A retrospective study of long-term tamoxifen users being put together in the United Kingdom may provide some information. A prospective study might take 20 years to answer the question."

Dr. Wolmark: "The issue of 5 versus 10 years in node-positive patients remains a valid research question. However, we at the NSABP have stopped tamoxifen at 5 years for our node-positive breast cancer protocols, based on the data from the node-negative population. I think this is the best information we have, and this decision has to be made by individual patients together with their physicians."

Dr. Jordan: "In my opinion, the question of 5 vs 10 years is almost a null hypothesis. Nobody really has done a valid comparison to determine an optimal tamoxifen duration. You won't be able to detect any difference between 5 and 10 years with clinical trials as they are set up because they are not large enough. An average size clinical trial would show no difference, just as the NSABP trial showed no significant difference.

"My early concern with the NSABP study was that it would show a significant detrimental effect after 10 years, with a large increase in recurrent disease, but that has not turned out to be the case."

11. How do you manage the menopausal symptomatology associated with tamoxifen use?

Dr. Jordan: "I would now like to ask our panel how they manage the postmenopausal symptoms that may occur with tamoxifen use, such as hot flashes and vaginal dryness. Dr. Wolmark, what are your specific recommendations for patients who develop these symptoms while taking tamoxifen?"

Dr. Wolmark: "The treatment of hot flashes in women taking tamoxifen can be problematic because of the need to limit estrogen use. We've tried various interventions such as Bellergal-S [belladonna, phenobarbital, and ergotamine tartrate], the low–dose Catapres [clonidine] patch, and vitamin E. And although these treatments have all been successful on occasion, none can be recommended as a standard intervention.

"When hot flashes are severe enough to significantly interfere with a woman's quality of life, then more aggressive therapy should be considered, including intravaginal estrogen preparations and even systemic estrogens. I want to make it very clear that I am not recommending systemic estrogens as an adjunct to tamoxifen to deal with symptoms. Rather, its use should be restricted to selected cases of women with severe acute symptoms."

Hot flashes are not all that common and may be attributed both to tamoxifen and to the fact that many postmenopausal women stop hormone replacement therapy once breast cancer is diagnosed

Ms. Langer: "Younger women on tamoxifen may find it especially difficult to cope when thrust into menopausal symptoms. The thoughtful oncologist will often give brief estrogen interventions to alleviate severe acute symptoms. It may not be commonly known in the medical community that this practice is acceptable, especially among primary care physicians who may be following these patients long term."

Dr. Osborne: "Luckily, hot flashes are not all that common and may be attributed both to tamoxifen and to the fact that many postmenopausal women stop hormone replacement therapy once breast cancer is diagnosed. Anecdotally, I have had success in a handful of patients using serotonin reuptake inhibitors such as venlafaxine (Effexor) at doses that are subtherapeutic for antidepressive activity."

Dr. Ragaz: "In my experience, women who increase their physical activity, through jogging or other regular exercise, often see a decrease in their hot flashes."

Dr. Jordan: "What about vaginal dryness? Dr. Osborne?"

Dr. Osborne: "Vaginal dryness is generally easily managed with use of vaginal creams. In a patient who is on tamoxifen, I have little fear of absorption of estrogen from the vagina. Short-term treatment of a few weeks is often effective, and you may not have to treat the patient again for months or even years."

Dr. Barakat: "Local applications of lubricating agents such as Replens or Astroglide gel may also help patients with vaginal dryness with sexual function."

Dr. Ragaz: "Some of our patients with vaginal dryness have reported benefits with use of over-the-counter lubricants containing primrose oil or jelly."

12. Should chemotherapy be added to tamoxifen or vice versa?

Dr. Jordan: "That concludes my own list of questions for the panel, and now I would like to put to them some questions that have been collected from the audience. The first concerns the use of adjuvant chemotherapy in patients taking tamoxifen and is addressed to Dr. Osborne."

Dr. Osborne: "I think there are still some uncertainties in this area, and there are ongoing clinical trials that should help to better define where we stand. But if you look at individual trials of premenopausal women, or the meta-analysis, in women who are getting chemotherapy, there doesn't seem to be much of an additional advantage for adding tamoxifen. It may be because many of these patients are already getting another endocrine therapy in the form of chemically induced ovarian ablation.

"The key question in older women is not whether you should add tamoxifen to chemotherapy, because in this group of patients tamoxifen is the standard agent. The question is whether you should add chemotherapy to tamoxifen. The majority of the studies don't show a survival advantage for the addition of chemotherapy to tamoxifen, although they do show a disease-free survival advantage. However, in the 3-arm NSABP trial, the arm containing doxorubicin/cyclophosphamide therapy did show a disease-free survival advantage in postmenopausal ER-positive women getting tamoxifen.

"Although the NSABP trial needs to be confirmed, I think we must conclude from the available evidence that in postmenopausal women there may be a slight advantage of adding a doxorubicin-containing regimen to tamoxifen, whereas in younger women, I'm not convinced of any advantage for the addition of tamoxifen to chemotherapy."

Dr. Ragaz: "The Oxford Overview analysis initially showed a slight benefit of tamoxifen added to chemotherapy in premenopausal patients, but in the latest review, this was not significant. I would caution, however, that in most of the studies in the overview, women had taken tamoxifen for only 2 years, and we now know that 5 years is more beneficial. So the overview may not fully answer the question. This question is being tested presently in the randomized, prospective Canadian NCI MA-12 study which is randomizing, in ER-positive premenopausal patients getting adjuvant chemotherapy, the survival impact of tamoxifen for 5 years against placebo after the completion of chemotherapy. Therefore the answer to this question will become available."

Misconceptions within the patient population can lead to potentially serious consequences, such as stopping a drug that will provide survival benefits

13. Should patients taking tamoxifen worry about the development of "fatty liver?"

Dr. Jordan: "A patient advocate from the Alamo Breast Cancer Foundation in San Antonio says that she has encountered several patients on tamoxifen who have developed "fatty livers," and knows of two women who have stopped taking tamoxifen because of this finding. She asks if any panel members have seen this in their patients, and is it a concern?"

Dr. Wolmark: "We have not seen that specific entity as a result of tamoxifen treatment in the NSABP trials. We are unaware of this not uncommon phenomenon of fatty replacement of the liver occurring as a result of therapy with tamoxifen."

Unknown physician from audience: "Fatty liver is a benign condition that is actually quite common if you look for it, particularly in women who are overweight or have mild diabetes. Breast cancer patients taking tamoxifen are closely monitored for possible metastases, including CT scans of the abdomen. In reading these scans, the radiologist may note a fatty liver. That's actually reassuring to the oncologist and the patient because it does not represent metastatic disease, and it's not a problem that progresses to chronic liver disease. It frequently goes away with time, weight loss, or diabetes control."

Dr. Jordan: "This illustrates how misconceptions within the patient population can lead to potentially serious consequences, such as stopping a drug that will provide survival benefits."

14. Does tamoxifen have a role in ductal carcinoma in situ (DCIS)?

Dr. Jordan: "The next question, from a medical oncologist at the Medical University of South Carolina, Charleston, asks whether the NSABP B-24 protocol will define the use of tamoxifen in noninvasive breast cancer. Dr. Wolmark?"

Dr. Wolmark: "The NSABP B-17 trial determined that in patients with noninvasive breast cancer (DCIS), lumpectomy with radiation provides better local ipsilateral control than does lumpectomy alone. The B-24 protocol will answer the question of whether adding tamoxifen to lumpectomy and radiation therapy in these patients will offer further improve in local control.

"Unfortunately, we don't have the data from that trial yet. But if tamoxifen and radiotherapy in every other situation has been better than radiotherapy alone in controlling local ipsilateral recurrence, we're certainly hopeful that will be the case for DCIS, where one of the things that we're trying to control is the subsequent occurrence of invasive cancer. But right now we don't know."

15. How long should a male breast cancer patient receive adjuvant tamoxifen?

Dr. Jordan: "Now we have a question from a male survivor of breast cancer who has been taking tamoxifen for 2½ years. He wants to know if the recommendation to stop tamoxifen after 5 years applies to male breast cancer patients as well. Dr. Osborne?"

Dr. Osborne: "Male breast cancer seems to behave, in many ways, just like the female counterpart. Since it is so uncommon, there are no large studies, as there are in female breast cancer, to address the question of duration. However, in a male breast cancer patient who is taking adjuvant tamoxifen after surgery and has never had disease recurrence, I would follow the same rules as in female breast cancer. And my opinion is that outside of a clinical study, the drug should be stopped at 5 years. There are no data to suggest that longer than 5 years is better."

16. What happens if a patient stops taking tamoxifen on her own?

Dr. Jordan: "A member of the audience notes that physicians can't always control what their patients do; they can only advise. The question is, what happens if a patient stops taking tamoxifen on her own just to see if certain symptoms go away? Dr. Osborne, can you answer that?"

Health food store products are a bit of a black box because you don't know exactly what the components are

Dr. Osborne: "I'm sure that this is common, and I've had a number of patients tell me they have stopped the drug for a couple of weeks to see if it relieved symptoms. To really make an impact on the serum drug levels, however, you would have to stop taking tamoxifen for at least several weeks.

"We don't know what effect, if any, there would be on breast cancer survival if tamoxifen was stopped for a longer period of time, say 3 to 6 months. If the drug was restarted, perhaps the impact would be minimal, maybe not even measurable. After all, it's a small period of time relative to the 5 years that the woman may be taking tamoxifen. So I think that if a patient came to me and said she had stopped for 3 months but then restarted, I would say she probably has nothing to worry about."

17. Is it safe for patients to use phytoestrogen products to treat menopausal symptoms associated with tamoxifen?

Dr. Jordan: "We have a question about how physicians should respond to patients on tamoxifen who want to try so-called natural estrogen products to relieve menopausal symptoms? Dr. Osborne, can you comment?"

Dr. Osborne: "Phytoestrogen products are being sold in health food stores as remedies for hot flashes, and although some of them may work, I have always been hesitant to suggest them to patients because of the uncertainty about what is in them. They could contain 'good estrogens' in the sense that they block the breast-cancer-promoting effects of the 'bad' natural estrogen produced by the body. Soy products, for example, contain estrogen, and it has been suggested that the high soy consumption in Asian countries may help account for the lower incidence of breast cancer in Asian women. But these health food store products are a bit of a black box because you don't know exactly what the components are."

Dr. Henderson: "Perhaps it is because I am from California, but I have seen a number of patients on tamoxifen who have sought relief of hot flashes with phytoestrogen preparations. In general, I feel that these are probably neither safer nor more harmful than short courses of estrogen, but I try to make certain that patients who use them are fully informed."

18. Why do the effects of tamoxifen last so long?

Dr. Jordan: "Another audience member from the Alamo Breast Cancer Foundation wants to know why, if tamoxifen is cytostatic rather than cytotoxic, it continues to work after it is stopped. I would like to comment first, and then I'll turn the question over to Dr. Osborne.

"Laboratory evidence suggests that, in addition to its cytostatic effects, tamoxifen does also have a cytocidal effect, killing off breast cancer cells, but tamoxifen may help control breast cancer in a variety of ways. It appears, for example, that tamoxifen may have a profound effect on angiogenesis, eradicating tumor cells by denying them a blood supply."

Dr. Osborne: "Just 1 year of tamoxifen therapy has been shown to reduce the risk of breast cancer recurrence 10 years later. So there seems to be some permanent effect. You don't have to kill the tumor cells to eradicate the tumor if you can stop tumor cell proliferation. Tumor cells continue to die off naturally, but the number of replacement cells is so large that the tumor grows bigger over time. If you can shut off that proliferation, which is what we think tamoxifen does, then you could eradicate all the tumor cells without directly killing any of them."

Dr. Jordan: "I think we have entered an age of uncertainty about how long to give tamoxifen. We have to trust the evidence emerging from clinical trials and reevaluate our previous model. However, it may be that the gains that we get in some patients with long-term tamoxifen use are offset by tamoxifen-stimulated growth in other patients. Patients are not all the same, and this is why we must have huge clinical trials to be able to answer the question."

Dr. Wolmark: "I would like to emphasize that just because we're recommending that tamoxifen be stopped at 5 years, it doesn't mean that stopping tamoxifen will cause the tumor to start growing again. That's not what's happening. Whatever benefit is accumulated over that 5 years continues through 10 years of follow-up. What the NSABP study has shown is that adding 5 extra years of tamoxifen therapy does not increase the benefit and, also, that there's no rebound effect, no increased incidence of recurrence after tamoxifen is stopped."

Dr. Jordan: "That concludes our discussion. I would like to thank the entire panel for their excellent contributions, and I would also like to thank PRR, Inc. for putting on this event. Our hope was to be able to convey to a broader community the idea that the benefits of tamoxifen should be rationally weighed against the toxicities that have been seen. From the perspective of the benefits, I think the panel as a whole would agree that they far outweigh any of the concerns that have been raised."

Appendix 1

Translational Research: Applying Laboratory Discoveries to Patient Care

V. Craig Jordan, PhD, DSc
Director, Breast Cancer Research Program
Robert H. Lurie Cancer Center
Northwestern University Medical School

The precise biological events that occur in the breast to cause cancer are currently unknown. However, research over the past 50 years has provided a remarkable insight into the working of the normal cell that has acted as a framework to understand the process of carcinogenesis. If we can understand the normal cell, then perhaps we can detect differences in a cancer cell and attempt to correct the change.

The course of human disease has been documented by the medical profession throughout this century. Cancer of the breast has the ability to spread through the body, and based on the principle of "seed and soil," the "seed," or metastases from the primary tumor in the breast, travel throughout the body in the blood and lymphatic systems to lodge in distant organs of preference (Figure 1). The metastasis finds the correct "soil" to continue growth. To survive, chemical signals are transmitted from the metastases that encourage the growth of new blood vessels toward the growing metastasis. This process is called angiogenesis. The blood vessels supply nutrients and oxygen to the dividing metastasis that enable the tumor to continue growth at the expense of the host. Ultimately, the spread and unregulated growth of metastases throughout the body will overwhelm the host.

Clinical research has allowed physicians to determine the degree of spread from the breast by examining the axillary lymph nodes for the microscopic presence of tumor. Patients are then classified as good prognosis (node negative for tumor) or poor prognosis (many lymph nodes containing tumor) (Figure 2). Twenty years ago, patients were treated with breast surgery alone in the belief that, because some patients would be cured, the wise strategy was to wait for a recurrence in those who were not cured, and treat these latter patients on recurrence or progression. Now, adjuvant treatment with

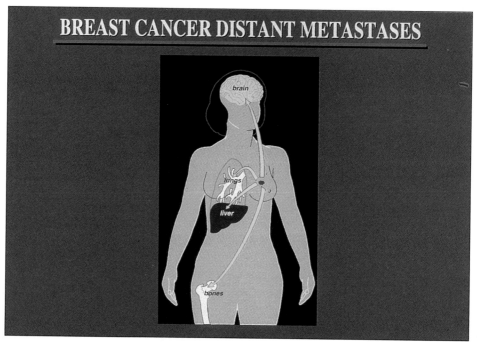

FIGURE I **Metastatic spread of breast cancer** The tumor cells travel through the blood and lymphatic system to lodge in organs of preference throughout the body, if not treated. The diagram illustrates some, but not all of the sites of potential metastatic spread. The metastases then continue to grow at the expense of the host in their new environment.

chemotherapy or tamoxifen is used after primary surgery to prevent recurrence by destroying unseen micrometastases around the body. This is the current strategy that is used to provide the best survival opportunity. The objective of all therapy with medicines is to destroy the metastases without harming the host; however, this is a difficult balance and toxicities occur because chemotherapy attacks both normal and cancer cells. However, the enormous success of tamoxifen, with its low incidence of side effects and targeted mode of action, has changed the strategy for treatment The current goal of research is to target vulnerable growth pathways in the tumor and to develop nontoxic treatments. The clinical description of human disease has been complimented by efforts in the research laboratory to understand the causes of mammary cancer in animals, under controlled conditions. Several principles have emerged that have ultimately provided an insight into the control and prevention of human disease. However, research does not travel in straight lines so that results and accomplishments in a laboratory model do not always provide solutions. Rather, in many instances, research only provides clues as to where to look for more information about human disease.

The description of the process of mammary carcinogenesis in laboratory animals has revealed targets to treat and to prevent the disease in women.

It has been known for most of this century that strains of mice can be bred that have a high incidence or a low incidence of mammary cancer. In the 1930's, a virus, called Bittners Milk Factor, was found to be transferred to the offspring in the mother's milk. This principle is unique to the mouse, and the virus, called mouse mammary tumor virus, is *not* generally believed to be involved in human disease. However, the virus has taught the research community a lot about carcinogenesis in the mouse. The gene has been thoroughly investigated and it is a research tool in molecular biology. The applications of the knowledge have been enormous and the success has opened the door for the discovery of "oncogenes" (ie, cancer causing genes).

In 1962, the Nobel laureate Professor Charles Huggins showed how a single dose of a polycyclic hydrocarbon derived from tar could produce mammary cancer in susceptible strains of rats. Chemicals had been linked to cancer all of this century, but the sensitivity and ease with which the tumors were produced in rats were the key. Mammary carcinogenesis was completely dependent on the age of the animals and the hormonal state, ie, the

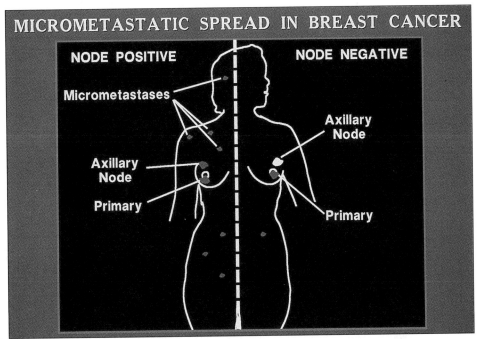

FIGURE 2 Classification of the stages of breast cancer as node positive and node negative The presence of microscopic tumor in the axillary lymph nodes is a marker of the spread of micrometastases throughout a patient's body.

FIGURE 3   **Mutation of oncogenes in the normal cell leads to an increase in stimulatory growth pathways**   The diagram shows only a few examples of the many dozens of reported changes. Growth factors like platelet derived growth factor (PDGF) can be increased and this activated oncogene product is called *sis*. Estrogen-receptor negative breast cancers have increased surface receptors that respond to epidermal growth factor (EGF). This is a normal stimulatory growth factor that is produced in many anatomic sites in the body, but the receptor also responds to the oncogenic stimulatory growth factor called transforming growth factor alpha (TGFα). The breast cancer cells produce an excess of the stimulatory growth factor that encourages growth through the EGF receptor know as *erb* B. A similar cell surface receptor called *HER-2/neu* is an oncogene product found in about 20% to 30% of poor prognosis breast cancers. Currently, attempts to target therapy to attack the *HER-2/neu* target have met with some success in the laboratory and there is encouraging clinical data to suggest that the oncogene is a marker for sensitivity to chemotherapy. The G proteins are signal transduction pathways that relay messages from the exterior to the interior of the cell. They operate as on/off switches. About 10% of breast cancers have a mutation at an oncogene product called *ras* that is stuck in the on position. Additionally, we know that the chemical carcinogens that produce mammary tumors in rats specifically mutate the *ras* gene.

presence or absence of the sex steroids estrogen and progesterone. However, some strains of rats are completely resistant to the chemical carcinogen. This again highlights the difference between laboratory animals and women. The animals are inbred to be vulnerable to the carcinogenic insult and it is now clear that the same process cannot readily happen in women. The human is outbred and not inbred, so, in general, we are not vulnerable to carcinogens and we survive through sophisticated repair mechanisms in our cells. Nevertheless, some principles have translated from the laboratory to the clinic. It is known from atom bomb survivors at Hiroshima and from adolescents who received radiation treatments for Hodgkin's disease that there is an increased susceptibility in young girls for radiation to initiate breast cancer. A significant radiation insult to young girls increases the risk for breast cancer in later life. This is also true for the young laboratory rat of the correct strain, whether the carcinogenic insult is radiation or a chemical. There is only a narrow window of time when the mammary gland is vulnerable to the initiation of cancer. However, it was found in the laboratory that female sex hormones are essential. Cancer does not occur if the animal has no ovaries. We also know that restricting the influence of the ovaries can have a profound effect on the development of breast cancer in humans. Men have less than 1% of the

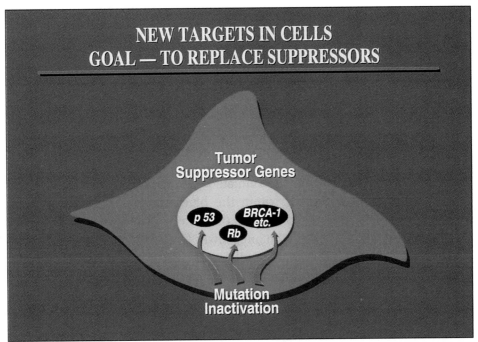

FIGURE 4 Tumor suppressor genes are proteins that function by restricting cell replication A mutation, or small change in the protein, will change its shape and it will not be able to perform its function as a cellular brake. The Rb or retinoblastoma protein was discovered to be responsible for the genetically transmitted cancer of the eye called retinoblastoma. Susceptible individuals are at genetic risk of having their low compliment of Rb destroyed by mutation of the tumor suppressor gene DNA. This destruction of the brake causes cancers in the affected individuals. The protein p53 is mutated in all different sorts of cancers and the unmutated protein appears to be a tumor suppressor gene. The breast cancer susceptibility gene BRCA-1 is mutated in high-risk individuals with a genetic family history of breast cancer. It is not known whether BRCA-1 is a tumor suppressor gene or a specialized inhibitory growth factor. (See Appendix 3)

incidence of breast cancer compared with women, and women who have an oophorectomy for medical reasons in their mid–30s generally have half the incidence of breast cancer in later life compared with women who have a natural menopause at 50. Therefore, it is believed that estrogen is intimately involved in the development and the growth of breast cancer.

But does estrogen cause breast cancer?

Laboratory studies have dissected the process of carcinogenesis into two stages: initiation and promotion. Initiation involves a genotoxic insult that alters the pattern of DNA, the blueprint for future generations of cells. The DNA can be altered by genotoxic chemicals or radiation, but in general the cell can quickly repair the damage before the imprint or mistake is made permanent in future generations of cells through rapid replication.

What controls the replication of cells and growth in general? Normal cells maintain their boundaries through a carefully regulated conversation with their neighbors. This is accomplished by a balance of negative and positive chemical messengers called growth factors that affect the cells locally. A stimulatory growth factor will instruct cells to divide when an injury needs to be repaired and an inhibitory growth factor will prevent the cells from growing further once tissue repairs are complete. Those chemicals that act as accelerators or brakes on the same cell where they are made are called autocrine growth factors, but if they affect an adjacent cell they are called paracrine growth factors.

The process of carcinogenesis is initiated by mutations of proto-oncogenes that lie buried and quiescent within the blueprint of our DNA. A proto-oncogene is converted to an oncogene that is a growth stimulator by either increasing the production of a mutant growth factor or its cell surface receptor (Figure 3). The cells' own growth mechanisms are dysregulated and respond to the hyperstimulation of growth messages.

However, an increase in accelerator growth signals is only one side of the story. Cells have regulator proteins within the nucleus that stop dysregulated growth. These are called tumor suppressor genes. The tumor suppressor gene can also be mutated so that the stop signal for replication in the cell is no longer recognized (Figure 4).

It is therefore clear that a very complex sequence of events must occur, and not be corrected by cellular repair mechanisms, before cancer is initiated. The mistake must be consolidated at an early stage to allow the cancer any hope of progressing to invasive disease. This event is, therefore, rarely successful. However, if initiation *is* successful, estrogen provides the fuel to drive the damaged cells through replication before the repair of mutations is complete. The mistakes to the DNA blueprint are copied faithfully in future

FIGURE 5 **The mutation of oncogenes or tumor suppresser genes by initiators of carcinogenesis acts to disrupt the integrity of the DNA** The damage is consolidated by rapid cycles of cell replication so the mistakes do not get repaired. Estrogen acts to promote and consolidate the carcinogenic insult that ultimately results in tumor formation.

generations to form a cancer cell. Estrogen allows the microfoci of deranged cancer cells to expand and they may even amplify their estrogen receptor population to maintain the growth response. Other tumor cell populations may develop new growth pathways by mutations of other growth regulator genes. The estrogen receptor will then become vestigial and redundant.

Cancer is characterized by genetic instability and the possibility of the mutant cell surviving at the expense of its female host can be unlimited. The diagrams illustrated in Figure 5 show the activation of oncogenes, the destruction of tumor suppressor genes by mutagens (chemicals or radiation), and finally the process of carcinogenesis being promoted to completion by estrogen. The malignant cell can then initiate disease progression by metastasizing in other parts of the body.

The knowledge of carcinogenesis has now promoted a focused evaluation of new therapeutic strategies to either prevent or at least localize breast cancer. Diligent laboratory research has made these opportunities possible and some of the strategies are illustrated in Figure 6. There is currently intense interest in developing a nutritional strategy to prevent cancer. The

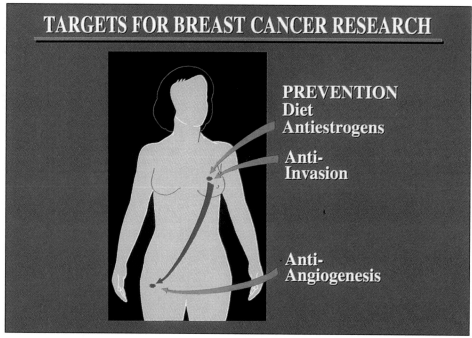

FIGURE 6 Strategies that are being evaluated to prevent breast cancer Lifetime nutritional factors may be important to prevent breast cancer, but tamoxifen is being tested in clinical trials in the United States, Britain, and Italy to block the promoting effects of estrogen. Additionally, drugs that prevent tumor invasion could prevent spreading. However, when malignant cells *do* spread to distant sites, then an antiangiogenic drug might prevent the formation of blood vessels and starve the metastasis. Without nutrients from the host, the tumor will die.

epidemiologic data points to a varying incidence of different cancers in different countries. Might it be the environment, or perhaps diet?

A whole host of dietary factors may be involved and laboratory research has identified several protective factors like antioxidants, phytoestrogens, and various fish oils that can alter carcinogenesis in animals. Similarly a high fat diet has been implicated in increased cancer risk. However, it is not easy to alter the lifestyle of the nation from conception to the grave to prove the role of nutrition in the development of cancer. Indeed it is well known that it is very difficult for our society to control food consumption in general. The antiestrogens, on the other hand, can be used in the context of clinical trials to answer a straightforward question: "Does 5 years of tamoxifen therapy prevent breast cancer in a woman with high risk?" That question is being addressed through nationwide clinical trials comparing tamoxifen treatment with a placebo (the tablet without tamoxifen). Biases are avoided by coding the treatments and observing the results only after years of data collection of the positive and negative effects of treatment. Without clinical trials, the question of the safety and worth of tamoxifen as a preventive cannot be answered. The alternative is the individual judgment of physicians to recommend treatment based on his or her prejudice or anecdotal experience. This was the method of medicine up to the 1960s and it should be prevented from returning so that our community remains protected.

The exciting possibility of prevention that is being tested in the tamoxifen trials does not end with tamoxifen, but with the results of the trials. The result will be the answer to the question "Can an *antiestrogen* prevent breast cancer with a minimum of side effects?" Already a spectrum of new antiestrogens and approaches to this research question are being positioned by the pharmaceutical industry so, by the turn of the century, numerous new antiestrogens will be benefiting from the information obtained with tamoxifen today.

The two other major research questions focus on the concept of restricting the spread of cancer when it occurs. New drugs are being developed that prevent malignant cells from destroying normal tissue around them. This process of destruction allows the micrometastasis to enter the blood and lymphatics in the breast and spread around the body. The chemicals secreted by the tumor cells that are called proteases and collagenases eat into the surrounding tissue in front of the malignant cell. The concept is like a snowblower eating into deep snow to create a path to the road: the drug target is the snow blower that can be stopped with a fallen branch jammed in the blades. Clearly these drugs could be used as preventives in high-risk women. If a tumor occurred in the breast it would not spread around the body and could be detected and completely cured by surgery.

The final point of attack is when the micrometastasis has found a suitable "soil" and needs to grow through unlimited access to nutrients from the host. If a strategy can be devised to stop angiogenesis, the process of obtaining a blood supply, then the micrometastasis will starve to death.

Conclusions

Overall, ideas developed in the laboratory are being rapidly translated into practical weapons to treat breast cancer. Only through continued research will our ability to control breast cancer be assured. It is essential to train and support a new generation of physicians interested in laboratory science and scientists interested in the control of breast cancer. It is people who make discoveries and it is people who can advocate new ideas to change the approach to a cure for breast cancer. The support of young investigators in centers of research excellence with a proven record of successful accomplishment is the best investment for the future of scientific discovery.

Appendix 2

How Does Tamoxifen Work?

V. Craig Jordan, PhD, DSc

There is no simple answer to the complex issue of the molecular events that not only cause tamoxifen to act as a targeted antitumor agent in the breast, but which also cause additional positive effects around a woman's body (Figure 1). A possible explanation must be divided into three different aspects: (1) the local antitumor actions of tamoxifen in breast cancer cells, (2) the peripheral antitumor actions of tamoxifen, and (3) the physiological actions of tamoxifen.

Local Antitumor Actions of Tamoxifen in Breast Cancer Cells

In the 20 years since Dr. Marc Lippman first showed that tamoxifen inhibits the growth of estrogen-receptor-positive breast cancer cells in culture, this model has been used extensively to dissect the molecular components of estrogen and antiestrogen actions. The molecular mechanism by which estrogen can control replication is illustrated in Figure 2.

A cascade of events in the cell is triggered by estrogen from the circulation which diffuses into the cell to bind to an estrogen receptor in the nucleus. The receptor complex becomes activated by changing its shape; two complexes are then believed to work in concert to activate estrogen-responsive genes composed of DNA. The genes are decoded by the transcription complex to make messenger RNA that makes a new protein in the cell cytoplasm. This process is called translation. Simply stated, the release of a trigger mechanism has the effect of making multiple new proteins that all have separate functions and, once orchestrated correctly, will convince the machinery of the cell to replicate itself through the duplication of DNA (the blueprint of the cell).

Some of the critical genes for replication are currently elusive, although the application of knowledge derived from the laboratory during the past decade has revolutionized our understanding of the molecular biology of cell replication. The key, though, is the trigger mechanism. If this can be blocked or immobilized, the cell will not divide on command.

Tamoxifen is a nonsteroidal antiestrogen that binds to the estrogen receptor but cannot produce the correct folding in the protein to switch on the ideal sequence of events that make specific replication proteins efficiently. The

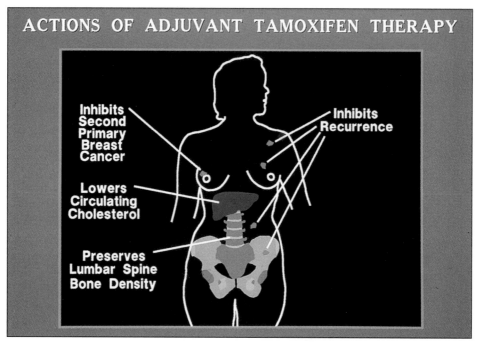

FIGURE 1 Target site-specific effects of tamoxifen in patients with breast cancer. Tamoxifen is proven to increase survival by preventing disease recurrence, and it is the only therapy that reduces the incidence of contralateral breast cancer. These effects can be considered to be antiestrogenic actions of tamoxifen. In contrast, tamoxifen maintains bone density and lowers circulating cholesterol in postmenopausal patients. These important physiologic effects may help to prevent osteoporosis and coronary heart disease in women at high risk for these diseases of the menopause.

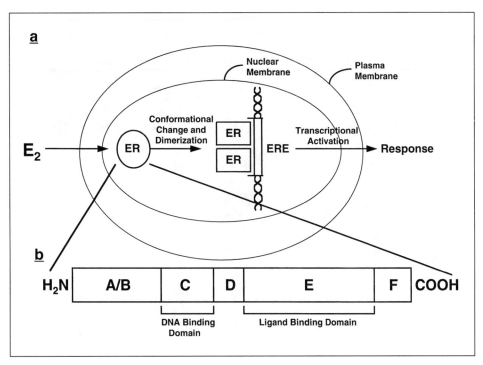

FIGURE 2 **(a) Estrogen-receptor mediated signal transduction pathway** Estradiol (E_2) diffuses through the cellular membranes to the nucleus where it binds to the estrogen receptor (ER). This induces a conformational change, causing the ER to dimerize and interact with the estrogen response element (ERE). Transcriptional activation occurs, resulting in a phenotypic response for a particular target cell. **(b) Organization of the ER indicating the five functional domains** They are subdivided into regions A/B, C, D, E, and F. Regions that contain the DNA-binding domain and the ligand-binding domain are shown.

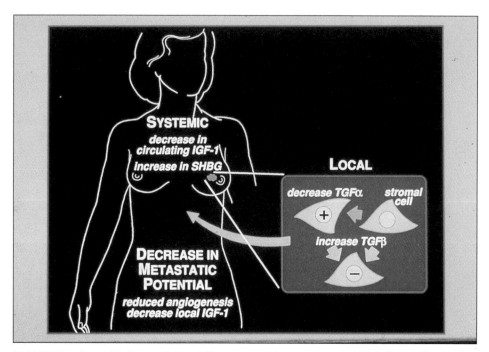

FIGURE 3   Overall effects of tamoxifen as an antitumor agent.   The effects of tamoxifen in a breast tumor [inset] are to decrease the secretion of stimulatory growth factors, such as transforming growth factor alpha (TGFα), and to increase the secretion of an inhibitory growth factor, such as transforming growth factor (TGFβ). TGFβ is known to inhibit the growth of estrogen receptor (ER)-negative cells, and it is believed that this is how tamoxifen can be effective in the patient with an estrogen-receptor-poor tumor. TGFβ functions as a paracrine growth factor, controlling the growth of an adjacent cell. Similarly, tamoxifen is thought to increase TGFβ production in the stromal cells in the tumor. The stromal cells act as a skeleton or support for the cancer cells in the tumor. Although these local antitumor effects may be essential, tamoxifen can also decrease the local and circulating levels of a stimulatory growth factor called insulin-like growth factor-1 (IGF-1). This growth factor stimulates the growth of both ER-positive and ER-negative tumors. Tamoxifen lowers the available level of circulating estrogen in a postmenopausal woman's body by increasing the level of sex hormones binding globulin (SHBG), a blood transport protein that binds estrogenic steroids. If the steroids remain bound in the blood, they cannot diffuse into the estrogen-receptor-positive tumor. Finally, tamoxifen may contribute to survival by decreasing tumor invasion and preventing angiogenesis, ie, the production of new blood vessels by the metastases.

cells cannot sustain cycles of replication and will remain quiescent as long as tamoxifen is present, blocking the receptors. The tamoxifen receptor complex will either initiate the death of the cells in the tumor or stop new cell replication. A breast tumor may decrease in size because most cells start to die as a result of tamoxifen therapy. Tumors go into remission because the cells necessary for the growth of the tumor cannot be replaced.

Usually tumors are composed of mixtures of both estrogen-receptor-positive and estrogen-receptor-negative cells (Figure 3). This "community" of cells help and support each other through the growth factor secretion so that some resistant cells can survive at the expense of their neighbors. Conversely, inhibitory growth factors secreted from estrogen-receptor-positive tumor cells in response to tamoxifen therapy can potentially control the growth of adjacent estrogen-receptor-negative cells. This stasis (inactivity) of growth for a mixed cell population could account for responses observed clinically in a few patients with "estrogen-receptor-poor" tumors.

The Peripheral Antitumor Actions of Tamoxifen

There are three potential points of attack that could be responsible for the survival advantages seen in patients treated with adjuvant tamoxifen therapy (Figure 3). Tamoxifen could reduce metastatic spread by:

• Reducing the production of estrogen-regulated proteases that are required to maintain invasion

• Reducing the circulating level and local production of stimulatory growth factors (for example, insulin-like growth factor [IGF]1) that might be essential to maintain the growth response of early micrometastases

• Reducing the angiogenic potential of micrometastases.

Each of these concepts has been noted in laboratory studies but it is unclear whether they contribute singly or together to the effectiveness of tamoxifen. It should be pointed out, though, that the associated antitumor actions would all support the overall direct antitumor effects of tamoxifen on the metastasis.

Physiological Actions of Tamoxifen

The actions of tamoxifen in the postmenopausal woman are a paradox. The ability to inhibit breast cancer growth is classified as an antiestrogenic action, whereas the action of tamoxifen on the level of circulating cholesterol and bone could be viewed as estrogenic. However, close examination of the actual effects shows that the changes produced by tamoxifen cannot be explained in these simple terms. Tamoxifen produces a selective estrogenic effect on postmenopausal bone. Similarly, the effect on cholesterol is to lower low-

Possible Mechanisms of Target-Site-Specific Action of Antiestrogens

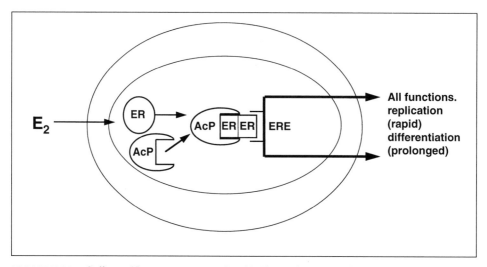

FIGURE 4A   Cell-specific accessory proteins (AcP) may be required to elicit the ER-mediated response. In a general model of estradiol (E_2) action, E_2 diffuses through the cellular membranes, interacts with the estrogen receptor (ER) and associates with a cell-specific AcP, allowing the E_2-ER complex to assume a favorable conformation and elicit a complete estrogenic response.

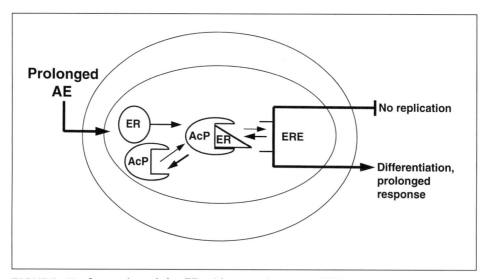

FIGURE 4B   Interaction of the ER with an antiestrogen (AE) may induce a variety of transcriptional responses, depending upon the availability of accessory proteins in a specific cell type. One hypothesis is that the AR-ER complex may induce a conformational change in the ER that does not allow a strong association with a required AcP; thus, an attenuated response is elicited, with differentiation but no replication.

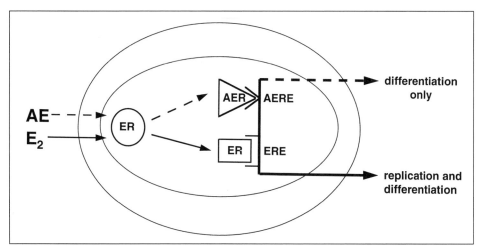

FIGURE 4C A second hypothesis involves specificity at the ERE. The AE-ER complex may interact specifically with distinct DNA sequences, antiestrogen response elements (AERE), to mediate differentiation but not replication. The diagram shows the AE (broken line) and the E_2 (solid line) going down separate pathways to produce select responses.

density lipoprotein cholesterol, but unlike estrogen, tamoxifen does not increase high-density lipoprotein cholesterol.

The most unusual effects are observed in the postmenopausal uterus. Tamoxifen produces estrogen-like symptoms in some women, but in others there is a complete antiestrogenic effect. There is a selective effect in the uterine cells of the majority of women. Stromal tissue of the endometrium is increased whereas the epithelium does not undergo hyperplasia. The reason for the target site-specific effects of tamoxifen around a woman's body is unknown. Current research is investigating the possibility that genes are selectively activated by the tamoxifen-estrogen receptor complex, or that groups of helper proteins that facilitate gene activation may only be found at some sites recognized as estrogen target tissues (see Figures 4A, 4B, and 4C). This is an area of intense scientific research that could provide vital information to develop new target site-selective antiestrogens in the future.

Appendix 3

Breast Cancer Susceptibility Gene BRCA-1

V. Craig Jordan, PhD, DSc

The past decade has witnessed a successful collaboration between epidemiology and molecular biology. Familial breast and ovarian cancer clusters have been documented that account for 10% to 15% of the annual incidence of breast cancer in the U.S. The gene responsible for susceptibility to this form of cancer is referred to as BRCA-1. This gene is mutated at different places in the germline. In hereditary breast and ovarian cancers, the growth of a tumor results from the loss of a normal allele. The fact that there are many potential sites of mutation makes the job of determining the precise sequence of the entire BRCA-1 gene in a woman time consuming and expensive. Nevertheless, absolute confirmation that an individual is carrying the mutated BRCA-1 gene dramatically alters the person's risk for breast and ovarian cancer compared to that of the general population This relationship is illustrated in Figure 1 and Figure 2. Women with a BRCA-1 mutation have an 80% cumulative risk of developing breast cancer by the age of 70. In contrast, women without a mutation have only an 8% cumulative risk of developing breast cancer. Women with a BRCA-1 mutation have a 44% cumulative risk of developing ovarian cancer compared with a 0.6% risk in women without a mutation.

A woman who has had one breast cancer has an increased risk of developing a second breast cancer in the other (contralateral) breast. Identification of a BRCA-1 gene mutation in a woman with breast cancer is associated with a nearly 50% risk of contralateral breast cancer by age 50 (Figure 3); in contrast, breast cancer survivors without BRCA-1 mutations have only a 7% to 10% risk of contralateral breast cancer.

Although the precise function of BRCA-1 is unknown, (Figure 4) exciting clues to its properties make research on the protein extremely important. The gene encodes an 1863 amino acid RING-finger protein (220-kD) which has led some to suggest that the protein functions as a tumor suppressor in the nucleus of the cell by blocking excessive gene activation. However, other research suggests that BRCA-1 is a secreted protein that belongs to the granin family. During pregnancy, the messenger RNA for BRCA-1 increases

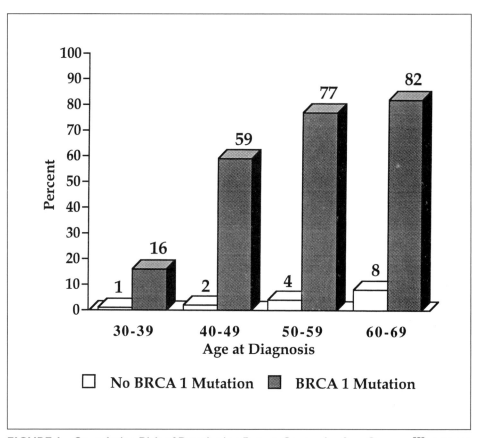

FIGURE I   Cumulative Risk of Developing Breast Cancer by Age Group   Women are divided according to presence or absence of a mutation in the BRCA-1 gene. Modified from Easton DF, Bishop DT, Ford D, et al: Genetic lineage analysis in familial breast cancer and ovarian cancer: Results from 214 families. *Am J Human Genetics* 52: 678-701, 1993 (with permission).

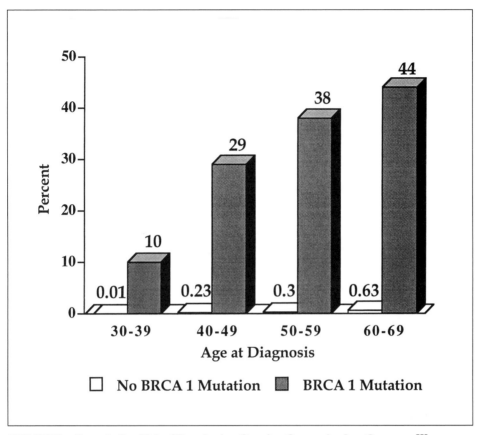

FIGURE 2   Cumulative Risk of Developing Ovarian Cancer by Age Groups Women are divided according to presence or absence of a mutation in the BRCA-1 gene. Modified from Easton DR, Bishop DT, Ford D, et al: Genetic lineage analysis in familial breast cancer and ovarian cancer: results from 214 families *Am J Human Genetics* 52:678-701, 1993 (with permission).

in breast epithelial cells; there are reports that the human and mouse protein is expressed in response to estrogen. By all indications, it appears that the protein is an inhibitory growth regulator or brake that is capable of preventing growth. Clearly, if this protein is mutated or damaged, the inhibitory function cannot be carried out and growth will become relentless. Most inherited BRCA-1 mutations produce truncated proteins that vary from 5% to 99% of the full-length protein. Whereas point mutations in BRCA-1 of sporadic tumors are very rare, complete somatic deletion of one allele of BRCA-1 occurs in approximately 50% of sporadic breast cancers. Further clinical risk factors are considered in Chapter 1.

There is currently no information about the therapeutic role of tamoxifen in women who test positive for BRCA-1 mutations. Information about the

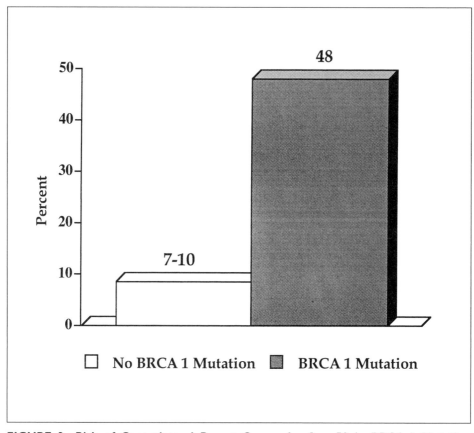

FIGURE 3 **Risk of Contralateral Breast Cancer by Age 50 in BRCA-1 Mutation Cancers**   Data from Ford D, Easton DF, Bishop DT, et al: Risk of cancer in BRCA-1 mutation cancers. *Lancet* 343:692-695, 1994 (with permission).

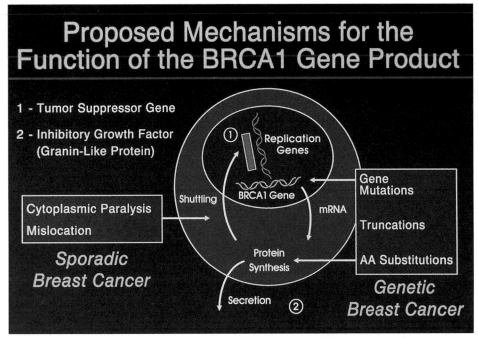

FIGURE 4 Proposed Mechanisms for the Function of BRCA-I Gene Product The BRCA-1 gene could be either (1) a tumor-suppressor gene blocking cell replication or (2) an inhibitory growth factor that is secreted. In genetic breast cancer, the gene is randomly mutated, leading to truncation or shortening of the protein. This will stop the protein from functioning. Alternatively, there may be single-point mutations that cause the miscoding of the protein. In sporadic breast cancer, there may be a mislocation of the BRCA-1 gene product so it is in the wrong place in the cell.

effectiveness of tamoxifen to reduce the incidence of early onset breast cancer is one of the primary goals of the prevention trials. Completion of these trials will provide some answers that will aid in the planning of additional studies in selected women. Tamoxifen has currently no role in protecting women from ovarian cancer, but again, this can only be evaluated when the results of the prevention trials are available.

For the future, it is possible that basic knowledge of the BRCA-1 and the much larger BRCA-2 proteins can herald a new era of therapeutics. If the proteins are only active in the breast and also selectively inhibit ovarian cancer, then new targeted therapies—which might maintain patients at risk in an inhibited state—will be possible. This maintenance treatment would be analogous to the diabetic who is successfully maintained on insulin injections for decades.

Suggested Reading

Komb A, Skolnick MH: Identification of the BRCA-1 breast cancer gene and its clinical implication, in DeVita VT, Hellman S, Rosenberg SA (eds): *Important Advances in Oncology*, pp 23-35. Philadelphia, Lippincott-Raven Publishers, 1996.

Appendix 4

How Are Drugs Developed?

Ruth O'Regan, MD
Fellow, Hematology/Oncology Division

V. Craig Jordan, PhD, DSc
Director, Breast Cancer Research Program
Robert H. Lurie Cancer Center
Northwestern University Medical School

The Western world is committed to, and profits from, a system of continuous change. A tenet of our society is "there must be a better way of achieving success." So it is with the development of medicines to treat disease. Citizens invest in the process by buying stock in the pharmaceutical industry, whose business goal is to discover new medicines to treat disease. Without the investment there would be very few drugs.

A Long, Costly Road

During this century, this process has been remarkably successful with the Western pharmaceutical companies, whose discoveries are initially protected by patent laws, providing society with virtually every new medicine that is used today. Regrettably, the process of discovery has no guarantee of success and depends on the professionals whose careers are dedicated to the search. It is, as a result, a long and very costly process, with hundreds of failures for every success. But the beneficiaries of success are the citizens who make discovery possible by investing in the process and the citizens who will live healthier and longer lives.

Nevertheless, there are legitimate concerns and criticisms about health care costs, but often the criticism results from a lack of understanding of how drugs are discovered and how much time and dedication is involved. Drugs do not come from the government or some company that accidentally finds an obscure plant or compound. They are discovered by trained individuals who must subject their discovery to the most rigorous of tests before it can be used to treat human disease.

The issue of drug costs was raised in a recent letter to *The Chicago Tribune* (Tuesday, August 6, 1996):

Vial Thoughts

Chicago—Lately, nearly every conversation that I have had with senior citizens has started with, or soon turned to, the high cost of senior health care. Singled out for the most heated comments have been the high prices of medication.

Almost always overlooked in these complaints has been the point that the expense of those life-sustaining chemical morsels is largely determined by the research effort that went into discovering and determining the utility of those magic little molecules that give these pills their efficacy—and, of course, the extensive safety checking that had to be done before they could go on the market.

The price of the chemical raw materials and the manufacture of the pills are not what makes them cost so much. If that were all that was involved, in most cases they would be dirt cheap.

It takes a lot of money to hire and equip labs, and when one considers those pills from a risk/benefit point of view, it's the biggest bargain we seniors ever got.

–Carl E. Moore
Emeritus Professor of Chemistry
Loyola University, Chicago

Clearly the synthesis, packaging, and distribution of a new medicine is not the important cost. The real expense is the cost of the hundreds, perhaps thousands of salaries for professionals whose technical skill have made a discovery possible and who have taken it from the bench to the bedside. Teams of synthetic organic chemists, who have spent most of their lives in training programs, initially have the task of making pure samples of novel compounds that will be passed on to the biologists who will test for the activity required. Thousands of compounds will be synthesized and tested, and the task of focusing on the correct new compound will take years. But the search does not end here. Several compounds are then selected, all with good activity, but the questions must be asked "Will the new drug be safe? Although we may be able to treat the disease, will the side effects be dangerous?"

The government sets down strict requirements that must be followed precisely before the FDA will permit clinical testing. Unfortunately, there is no exact way to predict harm to humans, but animal testing is an essential safeguard to protect citizens from the potential hazards of any new drug. For this reason, the toxicology testing usually takes many years and is extremely expensive. Highly skilled experts (pathologists and toxicologists), who have spent their lives training in the discipline, will evaluate all the available safety data from the animal studies before a new compound is chosen to test in a specific disease state.

Before a drug can be tested in humans it must be formulated. This involves the decision of how to give the drug to the patient. Questions must be addressed, such as "Do we make one tablet a day dosing? Should it be twice daily? Can we use injections? Should it be stored in the refrigerator, or away from light?" Pharmacists in industry play an essential role in drug development because without their skill any new medicine may be unacceptable to a patient or may lose its effectiveness too quickly. Only clinical trials will prove how skilled the industrial pharmacists have been.

Additionally, before the drug goes into clinical trial, a method of large-scale synthesis must be developed and a chemical manufacturing plant designed. It is one thing for a lone chemist to make a few teaspoons of a drug in the laboratory—this may take a week or so. It is, however, an entirely different matter to make tons of the new drug. All the truckloads of raw materials must be checked for purity; then the *final* product must be free of any impurities. Quality control is an essential and ongoing part of the drug manufacturing industry and this is strictly monitored by the government. Still, the drug is not yet ready for sale. The government has to be convinced that the drug is safe and that it works. The process can take many years.

The government sets down strict requirements that must be followed precisely before the FDA will permit clinical testing

Clinical testing of new drugs for cancer is divided into three phases (I, II, and III). The objective and rationale for each phase in the process of drug development is explained briefly in the following sections. Each of the testing phases is performed under the strictest requirements laid down by the FDA, and the pharmaceutical company is usually required to organize and to pay for the testing. Additionally, all experiments, all side-effects, and measures of response must be available for scrutiny by panels of experts at the FDA. Precise recordkeeping is an absolute requirement for the approval of any drug.

Phase I Trials

The objective of a phase I trial is to determine the relationship between toxicity of a drug in question, often an experimental agent, and to determine a dose schedule. Phase I studies are usually conducted in previously treated patients. However, they may be conducted in untreated patients provided no other therapeutic options exist. The organ systems expected to be targets of toxicity for the study drug should be competent or the data obtained will not be relevant in less debilitated patients. Phase I studies are not targeted at specific malignancies, and response of the malignancy to the study drug is not a major endpoint. However, response rates seen in certain malignancies may pave the way for phase II studies of this agent in this malignancy. The endpoints in phase I studies are to determine the toxicity of a given agent and to ascertain the maximum tolerated dose in order that a dose schedule for phase II studies can be determined.

The starting dose of the study drug is one that is not expected to produce serious toxicity in any patient. It is usually determined as a fraction of the lethal dose in animal studies. A certain number of patients, usually less than ten, are treated at this first dose level. If this dose is tolerated, it is then escalated in subsequent patients according to a series of preplanned steps. One common method treats a second group of patients at twice the dose of the dose used in the first group. A third group is then treated at a dose 67% greater than the second group, a fourth group at a dose 33% greater than the dose used in the third group, and so on until the dose-limiting toxicity is reached. Obviously, toxicity in each group must be below a certain level for dose escalation to occur in the next group.

The phase II dosage is usually the highest dose where the incidence of dose-limiting toxicity is less than 33%. It is important to point out that doses are not escalated in the same patient due to the risk of cumulative toxicity. More precise methods of dose escalation involve the use of the drug's serum level to determine further dosage. The number of patients required and the duration of a phase I trial may be huge, depending on how high the maximum dose is above the starting dose.

Phase II

Once the maximum tolerated dose is determined, the drug can be entered into phase II studies in malignancies where it has shown the most activity. The objective of phase II studies is to identify tumor types where a drug seems most active. Thus, the endpoint of a phase II study is the response of a certain tumor to a study drug. A large number of patients are needed to evaluate a response accurately. The study drug should first be tested in patients with malignancies most likely to have a favorable response. The most accurate information is obtained in patients with good overall performance status, minimal disease, and minimal prior treatment. In patients with a poor performance status and extensive prior treatment, it is often not possible to give the full desired dose. In addition, a lack of activity in such patients does not necessarily indicate a similar outcome in other patients. In malignancies known to be poorly sensitive to other treatments, it is reasonable to enroll untreated patients on phase II studies.

Phase II evaluation is not appropriate when treatment with curative potential is available. The results of phase II studies may unfortunately be misleading (either overly optimistic or unduly disappointing), as the studies are not randomized and the treatment outcomes are compared with historical controls. As a result, specific statistical methods are available to determine the required size and duration of phase II trials, based on likely response of the malignancy to the study drug. Prior to study commencement, the total number of patients necessary to achieve a certain response is ascertained. Of this total number, a proportion are analyzed early in the study to ensure that the desired response rate is being achieved. If the response rate is adequate in the initial group of patients, enrollment continues until the total number of patients is reached. This second group of patients is essential to estimate the true activity of the drug. If the desired response rate is not seen in the initial small group of patients, the trial is ended prematurely. The total number of patients required depends on the precision of the estimated response rate. The larger the number of patients, the more accurate the estimate of the response rate.

Quality of life aspects are becoming increasingly important as better methods of measurement are available

Phase III Trials

Once a study drug has demonstrated desired response rates in a given cancer compared with historical controls, it must be randomized against current standard therapies or practices. The objective of these phase III studies is to determine the effects of this new treatment relative to either the natural history of or standard therapies for the malignancy in question. Phase III studies may also compare a drug felt to have similar efficacy to the standard treatment to determine if the study drug is associated with less morbidity than the standard therapy. All patients eligible for a phase III study should be able to tolerate the allocated treatment. Results obtained in a phase III trial should be of such importance that they can be applied on a national and/or international basis.

The major endpoints of phase III trials are measures of patient welfare. Two such endpoints are survival and quality of life. Response rate is more of a subjective measurement, as it does not directly translate into a survival benefit and consequently improved patient welfare. Quality of life aspects are becoming increasingly important as better methods of measurement are available.

In phase III studies, patients are randomized to different treatments. As mentioned previously, comparison of results with historical controls is associated with considerable bias. Randomization significantly reduces bias. Patients may be randomized to study treatment or current standard therapy, which may be standard drug or no treatment. In a stratified randomized trial, patients are selected prior to randomization according to specific well identified risk factors. This ensures equal distribution of patients with regard to these risk factors and decreases the chance of gross imbalances that cannot be adjusted for at the end of the study. In a crossover study, a patient receives both the study drug and the control drug at different time intervals; therefore, patients act as their own control. Such studies are limited by a number of factors, including a change in the patient's condition over time. Factorial designs randomize patients to two different therapies initially and then subsequently to a further two therapies. The objective of such a study is to answer two questions for the "price" of one. Large numbers of patients are needed in these studies and the initial two treatments must have no effect on the second treatments and vice versa.

Size and duration of phase III trials are based on study objectives and endpoints. Follow-up must be specified clearly. Studies may be terminated prematurely due to unforeseen problems or greater-than-expected differences between the arms of the study. Target sample sizes are essential to ensure that the study is feasible and to determine when to stop accrual in the absence of premature termination. If too few patients are enrolled, the results may be either ambiguous or erroneous.

Significance of the Size of the Trial

It should be possible to accrue the desired sample size in a reasonable length of time. Determination of sample size is based on the assumption that, at the conclusion of the trial, a statistical significance test will be performed comparing the treatment groups with regard to the primary endpoint. The study will have a null hypothesis—for example, that the study drug results in improved survival when compared with control treatment—which will be either accepted or rejected at the end of the study. Through statistical means it will be determined whether the study drug is significantly better than the control drug. The significance level used in most studies is only five chances in 100, which means if the study drug is truly better than the control drug, the probability of not noting this difference is only 0.05. The number of patients enrolled dictates the likelihood of a truly significant result. If few patients are enrolled, the differences between the outcome with the study drug as compared with the control drug must be extreme to be significant. When greater numbers of patients are enrolled, smaller differences in outcome become significant at the 0.05 level. Therefore, to detect small differences between two groups, huge numbers of patients need to be enrolled, which may take many years. Tables are available which dictate how many patients need to be enrolled on both arms based on likely difference between the arms of treatment. All phase III trials should be large enough to detect a 20% difference between the groups. Interim analysis should be done only by the data monitoring committee and should be ignored unless noted differences are significant at the 0.0025 level.

At the end of phase III studies, if the study drug does indeed show a significant benefit in a particular malignancy, it will usually be approved for general use in that malignancy. Regrettably, these clinical trials can take a great many years to accomplish, and many drugs are abandoned along the way because they are either too toxic or do not have enough activity to be better than existing drugs.

After FDA Approval

Once a new drug is approved by the FDA committees for a particular indication, a company can advertise the approved claim. A company cannot make claims outside approved uses. For example, if a new drug is proved to be useful to treat advanced breast cancer, a company cannot advertise or imply, for example, that it should be used for adjuvant treatment of node-negative breast cancer. This is to protect the public from unforeseen problems. This is why there have to be clinical trials—to look for the good and the bad effects.

The number of patients enrolled in a clinical trial dictates the likelihood of a truly significant result

A pharmaceutical company is required to invest in clinical testing to provide evidence for the desired FDA approval. The process is exemplified by the development of tamoxifen (Nolvadex), which has been the only approved antiestrogen on the market in the United States since 1978. No other company was willing to make the investment to make alternatives available because it was generally believed that the research investment would not be useful. All the attention was focused on chemotherapy. However, through the clinical trials process, there has been a revolution in treatment that has dramatically improved the prognosis for women with breast cancer. The commitment of the manufacturers to provide millions of free tablets to the clinical trials community over the past 2 decades has resulted in the additional FDA approvals noted in Chapter 4. The work was completed, through National Cancer Institute-approved experimental protocols, by national organizations of physicians called the National Surgical Adjuvant Breast and Bowel Project (NSABP), the Eastern Co-Operative Oncology Group (ECOG), and the Southwest Oncology Group (SWOG). Thousands of physicians and health care professionals volunteered their time over decades to prove whether the best ideas for cancer treatment could provide benefit for their patients. Thousands of women with breast cancer made a commitment that they would participate to help themselves and future generations.

The key is that the driving force in this remarkable story were the physicians and scientists, not the companies. The clinical researchers spotted the potential for success in providing help for breast cancer patients, devised the clinical protocols, and committed themselves to the process of clinical investigation. Without this voluntary commitment there would have been no further FDA approvals for Nolvadex.

Generics

It is always stated that if a drug becomes generic it will be cheaper. This is true, but the reason it is true is important. The major pharmaceutical companies discover drugs and are required to shoulder the responsibility for their safety and to prove they work in patients. The investment costs hundreds of millions of dollars and it takes about a decade to complete the process. A patent protects the company so it can make the investment and effort and allows the company time to reclaim the overall costs in sales. Without patents and the power of the courts, no one would invest in drug discovery because someone else would steal the idea. If this was the situation, no drugs would be developed.

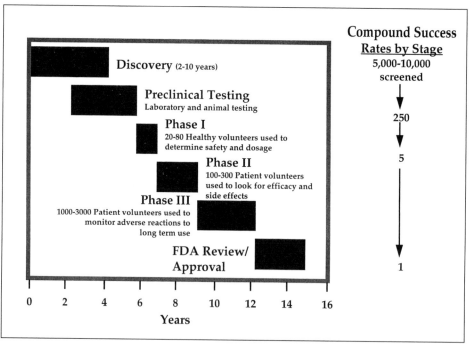

FIGURE 1   Drug discovery process to establish one new product that is FDA approved   For every new drug available, it is estimated that 5,000 to 10,000 new compounds need to be screened in the laboratory. Adapted from Pharmaceutical Research and Manufacturers of America: *PhRMA industry profile 1996: Opportunities and challenges for pharmaceutical innovation.* Washington, 1996.

In contrast, a company that makes generic drugs has no commitment to new drug discovery and testing, so the price only reflects the much smaller cost of synthesis and distribution.

Without our commitment to the process of change, there would be no medicines available to treat breast cancer. The patent laws secure progress, but it is important to appreciate that the process has not stopped with tamoxifen. "It is only the end of the beginning," as Winston Churchill said in 1942.

The success of tamoxifen has encouraged new ideas and initiatives that would never have been considered 20 years ago. At that time, no one was interested, but success breeds success. The profits from the success of Nolvadex have been reinvested to develop new drugs to treat breast and also prostate cancer (a disease that kills as many men as breast cancer does women). This commitment provides a choice of novel treatment strategies for both the physician and the patient. The development of tamoxifen as the leading cancer medicine has taken 30 years from concept to reality, so it is perhaps valuable to illustrate the time and cost of new drug development and the changes that are taking place in treatment practice. A time scale and cost estimate for the next generation of new drug development is shown in Figure 1.

Conclusion

In summary, it is clear that the inventiveness of Western society has provided enormous advantages for its citizens. However, the process of drug discovery and development takes years to accomplish safely and requires the investment of billions of dollars. Success depends upon the skill of individual scientists and physicians who have already dedicated much of their working lives being trained for the opportunity to contribute to the process of drug discovery and development. There are no shortcuts or quick ways to guarantee success. Nevertheless, as Carl E. Moore stated, "When one considers those pills from a risk/benefit point of view, it's the biggest bargain we seniors ever got."

Appendix 5

Y-ME Hotline: The Most Frequently Asked Questions About Tamoxifen

Y-ME is a national breast cancer organization headquartered in Chicago that serves hundreds of thousands of American women who have been diagnosed with breast cancer. Y-ME operates a hotline staffed to respond to questions concerning breast cancer diagnosis, treatment, and recovery. It provides educational meetings and support groups throughout the country, including educational workshops for the lay public, special programs for teenage girls, and a wig and prothesis bank. Y-ME publishes a bi-monthly newsletter as well as pamphlets targeting special audiences, such as single women or male partners of breast cancer patients. Many of Y-ME's services are also available in Spanish. Y-ME promotes the psychosocial needs of people with breast cancer and encourages women to be active participants in their medical care.

The ten most frequently asked questions about tamoxifen on the Y-ME hotline follow:

How long do I have to take tamoxifen?

This is a matter between you and your doctor. The standard duration of tamoxifen treatment in all US clinical studies is 5 years. Nevertheless, many patients have taken tamoxifen for more than 5 years and clinical trials are testing the value of indefinite tamoxifen treatment.

The National Cancer Institute has issued a Physicians' Alert stating that, for node-negative patients, 10 years of tamoxifen provides no greater benefit than 5 years. However, these results are based on the recurrences of patients in only one clinical trial; many in the clinical trial community believe that more information is needed. In fact, clinical trials conducted in England are addressing the issue of duration of tamoxifen therapy by recruiting 20,000 women who have stopped tamoxifen at various times to determine the risks and benefits in large patient populations.

Table 1

Percentage of Women Who Reported an Adverse Side Effect in the NSABP-14 5-Year Tamoxifen Trial (20 mg Daily) Vs Placebo

Both pre-and postmenopausal women participated in the study. These are the only side effects noted by the nearly 3,000 women involved in the trial. It should be recognized that all side effects were not experienced by all women.

Adverse Effect	Nolvadex (n = 1424)	Placebo (n = 1420)
Hot flashes	63.9%	47.6%
Weight gain (> 5%)	38.1%	40.1%
Fluid retention	32.4%	29.7%
Vaginal discharge	29.6%	15.2%
Nausea	25.7%	23.9%
Irregular menses	24.6%	18.8%
Weight loss (> 5%)	22.6%	18.0%
Skin changes	18.7%	15.3%
Increased BUN	18.1%	20.2%
Diarrhea	11.2%	14.0%
Increased SGOT	4.8%	2.8%
Increased alkaline phosphatase	3.0%	4.6%
Vomiting	2.1%	1.7%
Increased bilirubin	1.8%	1.2%
Increased creatinine	1.7%	1.0%
Thrombocytopenia*	1.5%	1.2%
Leukopenia**	0.4%	1.1%
Thrombotic events		
Deep vein thrombosis	0.8%	0.3%
Pulmonary embolism	0.4%	0.1%
Superficial phlebitis	0.3%	0.0%

*Defined as a platelet count of < 100,000/mm3

**Defined a white blood cell count of < 3,000/mm3

What are the side effects of tamoxifen therapy? Are they temporary or permanent?

There are a variety of minor side effects with tamoxifen and these should be discussed with your doctor. A comparison of side effects in placebo-controlled trials is illustrated in Table 1. The most common concern is postmenopausal symptoms. A minority of patients may suffer severe symptoms, but these will diminish with time. Some side effects, such as hot flashes, occur more frequently in younger women. Less than 5% of women stop tamoxifen because of side effects. Postmenopausal women should be aware that there is a modest increase in the detection of endometrial cancer in women who are taking tamoxifen. In general, one postmenopausal woman in 1000 will develop endometrial cancer each year. In postmenopausal women who take tamoxifen, the rate is two women who may have endometrial cancer diagnosed per 1000 per year. Any signs of vaginal spotting or bleeding should be reported to your doctor and followed up with a gynecologic examination [see Chapters 9 and 10].

Tamoxifen is the single most effective agent for the adjuvant treatment of breast cancer in postmenopausal women

How does tamoxifen work?

Tamoxifen has target site-specific actions. The drug acts as an antiestrogen to block breast cancer growth, but it also has an estrogenic effect to help maintain bone density and to decrease circulating cholesterol. Prolonged (5 years or more) use of tamoxifen is associated with a decrease in myocardial infarction (heart attacks). The way tamoxifen works as an antibreast cancer drug depends principally on its ability to block the growth effects of estrogen in the breast cancer. A majority of breast cancers contain estrogen receptors (locks) that bind estrogen (keys) in a woman's body. The estrogen fits the estrogen receptor in the tumor cell and turns on all of the reactions necessary to instruct the cell to divide. As a result, the tumor grows relentlessly with estrogen as the fuel. Tamoxifen binds to the estrogen receptor and blocks the ability of estrogen by stopping estrogen binding. It blocks the estrogen receptor—blocks the lock—as long as the drug is taken. Tamoxifen cannot switch on the proper mechanism to instruct the tumor to grow, so the cells die and the tumor shrinks.

Another way to understand the different effects that tamoxifen can produce around a woman's body is to view it as a programmed elevator key: the estrogen makes the elevator stop at all the floors, while the tamoxifen key only allows stops at some of the floors. Estrogen stimulates all sites around a woman's body *including* the breast cancer but tamoxifen stimulates all the sites *except* the breast cancer.

What happens if I don't take tamoxifen or stop taking it?

Forgetting to take the medication once in a while is not a cause for concern. Although 20 mg daily (one 20-mg tablet or two 10-mg tablets) is recommended, there is usually sufficient tamoxifen in the blood to protect you if tablets are forgotten.

Tamoxifen works as an anticancer agent if the drug is present to suppress the tumor. Without the drug, estrogen can reactivate the growth mechanism.

How should I monitor myself for side effects and problems?

The most important method is simply to report any major changes in your normal activities to your physician or health care professional. Tamoxifen is remarkably free from serious side effects, but it is often tempting to blame tamoxifen for problems normally associated with menopause or aging.

The side effects of tamoxifen are listed in Table 1. It is unlikely that an individual will experience all or even most of these side effects. This list includes symptoms from thousands of different women over many years. The single most important concern is the early detection of endometrial cancer [see Chapters 9 and 10]. If you experience any vaginal spotting or bleeding after menopause, you should tell your physician, who will then order a full gynecological examination.

How effective is tamoxifen?

Tamoxifen is the single most effective agent for the adjuvant treatment of breast cancer in postmenopausal women. Each woman will respond differently, depending upon the type and stage of breast cancer. However, the Overview Analysis of clinical trials convincingly demonstrates a survival advantage for women who take tamoxifen. On average, this can translate to a year or two more of life for women taking tamoxifen compared with women not taking tamoxifen. Tamoxifen is the only therapy that reduces the incidence of breast cancer in the other breast and also reduces the risk of local recurrence of breast cancer in the affected breast in women treated with lumpectomy and radiotherapy.

Where can I get tamoxifen at a reasonable price?

The price of tamoxifen has remained remarkably stable for the past 10 years. It is controlled in the United States through patent protection. More-over, Zeneca Pharmaceuticals believes that no woman who needs Nolvadex should be denied the drug because of her economic circumstances. Truly needy women can apply through their physicians to Zeneca's assistance program. Between 1978 and 1996, Zeneca provided more than $114 million worth of tamoxifen to needy patients.

Although tamoxifen works most effectively in patients with estrogen-receptor-positive disease, estrogen-receptor-poor patients can also benefit

Should I take tamoxifen if I'm ER-negative or premenopausal?

Tamoxifen is more effective in some circumstances than in others. Although tamoxifen works most effec-tively in patients with estrogen-receptor-positive dis-ease, "estrogen-receptor-poor" patients can also bene-fit. The point where the tumor is described as estro-gen-receptor-positive or -negative varies from place to place. For example, most laboratories have used a value of 10 femtomoles/mg protein as their cut-off point; values greater than 10 are considered estrogen-receptor-positive and those less than 10 are considered negative. In San Antonio, however, the cut-off point is 3 femtomoles/mg protein and the new techniques of immunocy-tochemistry do not have a quantitative scale at all. Therefore, it is best to consider patients as estrogen-receptor-rich or -poor.

Clinical trials with node-positive breast cancer patients over age 50 have noted that estrogen-receptor-poor patients have a survival advantage after taking tamoxifen. Although most physicians would follow the consensus guidelines that only node-positive patients with receptor-rich tumors should be given tamoxifen, the FDA-approved indications do not rule out tamoxifen for receptor-poor patients with node-positive disease.

The above situation contrasts with node-negative disease and premeno-pausal patients. Tamoxifen is FDA-approved for the adjuvant treatment of pre- and postmenopausal node-negative patients with estrogen-receptor-rich pri-mary tumors. Tamoxifen is also approved for the treatment of patients who are premenopausal with Stage IV (advanced) estrogen-receptor-positive breast cancer.

Can I get pregnant while on tamoxifen?

Tamoxifen should not be given to a woman who is known to be pregnant because of the concern about possible birth defects and harm to the fetus. Women who are of reproductive age *must* use barrier contraception to prevent pregnancy. Premenopausal women who take tamoxifen are at risk for pregnancy. Women who may wish to conceive after a diagnosis of breast cancer should consult their physicians because tamoxifen should not be prescribed. If a woman chooses to become pregnant after a course of tamoxifen, the drug should be stopped for up to six months before pregnancy is considered.

How is tamoxifen different than chemotherapy?

Tamoxifen is generally classified as an antiestrogen rather than a chemotherapy. In general, cytotoxic chemotherapy attacks all dividing cells in a woman's body, not just the cancer cells. As a result, chemotherapy is associated with a high level of toxic side effects. In contrast, tamoxifen does not have dangerous effects on normal cells, but it does stop the growth of tumors. It causes death in the tumor cells but does not injure other tissues. Side effects of tamoxifen are very low compared with any of the cytotoxic chemotherapies.

For additional information about Y-ME, please write to:
Y-ME
212 W. Van Buren, 4th Floor
Chicago, IL 60607-3908

Fax: 312-986-8338

National hotline: 1-800-221-2141
Spanish-language hotline: 1-800-986-9505 (M-F, 9-5, CST)

Appendix 6

Recommended Further Reading and References for Physicians and Scientists

Books

Harris J, Lippman M, Morrow M, Hellman S (eds): *Diseases of the Breast.* Philadelphia, Lippincott-Raven, 1996.

Wisemen H: *Tamoxifen: Molecular Basis of Use in Cancer Treatment and Prevention.* Chichester, John Wiley & Sons, 1994.

Jordan VC: *Long Term Tamoxifen Treatment for Breast Cancer.* Madison, Wisconsin, University of Wisconsin Press, 1994.

Lindsay R, Dempster DW, Jordan VC: *Estrogens and Antiestrogens.* Philadelphia, Lippincott-Raven, (in press).

Reviews in Refereed Journals

Gradishar WJ, Jordan VC: The clinical potential of new antiestrogens. *J Clin Oncol* (in press).

Assikis VJ, Neven P, Jordan VC, Vergote I: A realistic clinical appraisal of tamoxifen and endometrial carcinogenesis. *Eur J Cancer* 32A:1464–1476,1996.

Assikis VJ, Jordan VC: Gynecological effects of tamoxifen and association with endometrial cancer. *Int J Gyn Obstet* 49:241-257, 1995.

Jordan VC, Gradishar WJ: Molecular mechanisms and clincial potential of new antiestrogens. *Molecular Aspects of Medicine* (in press).

Bilimoria M, Assikis VJ, Jordan VC: Should adjuvant tamoxifen be stopped at 5 years? *The Cancer J from Sci Am* 2:140-150, 1996.

Index